Surgical Conditions of the Diaphragm

Editor

ERIN A. GILLASPIE

THORACIC SURGERY CLINICS

www.thoracic.theclinics.com

Consulting Editor
VIRGINIA R. LITLE

May 2024 • Volume 34 • Number 2

ELSEVIER

1600 John F. Kennedy Boulevard • Suite 1800 • Philadelphia, Pennsylvania, 19103-2899

http://www.thoracic.theclinics.com

THORACIC SURGERY CLINICS Volume 34, Number 2
May 2024 ISSN 1547-4127, ISBN-13: 978-0-443-12875-2

Editor: John Vassallo (j.vassallo@elsevier.com)
Developmental Editor: Anita Chamoli

Thoracic Surgery Clinics (ISSN 1547-4127) is published quarterly by Elsevier Inc., 360 Park Avenue South, New York, NY 10010-1710. Months of publication are February, May, August, and November. Business and editorial offices: 1600 John F. Kennedy Boulevard, Suite 1800, Philadelphia, PA 19103-2899. Periodicals postage paid at New York, NY, and additional mailing offices. Subscription prices are $434.00 per year (US individuals), $100.00 per year (US students), $487.00 per year (Canadian individuals), $100.00 per year (Canadian students), $225.00 per year (international students), $524.00 per year (international individuals). For institutional access pricing please contact Customer Service via the contact information below Foreign air speed delivery is included in all Clinics' subscription prices. All prices are subject to change without notice. **POSTMASTER:** Send address changes to Thoracic Surgery Clinics, Elsevier Health Sciences Division, Subscription Customer Service, 3251 Riverport Lane, Maryland Heights, MO 63043. **Customer Service (orders, claims, online, change of address): Telephone: 1-800-654-2452 (U.S. and Canada); 314-447-8871 (outside U.S. and Canada). Fax: 314-447-8029. E-mail: journalscustomerservice-usa@elsevier.com (for print support); journalsonlinesupport-usa@elsevier.com (for online support).**

Reprints. For copies of 100 or more, of articles in this publication, please contact Commercial Rights Department, Elsevier Inc., 360 Park Avenue South, New York, NY 10010-1710. Tel: 212-633-3874; Fax: 212-633-3820; E-mail: reprints@elsevier.com.

Thoracic Surgery Clinics is covered in *MEDLINE/PubMed (Index Medicus), EMBASE/Excerpta Medica, Science Citation Index Expanded (SciSearch®), Journal Citation Reports/Science Edition,* and *Current Contents®/Clinical Medicine.*

Contributors

CONSULTING EDITOR

VIRGINIA R. LITLE, MD
Chief of Thoracic Surgery, St. Elizabeth's
Medical Center, Professor of Surgery, Boston
University, Brighton, Massachusetts

EDITOR

ERIN A. GILLASPIE, MD, MPH, FACS
Associate Professor with Tenure, Chief,
Division of Thoracic Surgery, Creighton
University Medical Center CHI Health, Omaha,
Nebraska

AUTHORS

ALEJANDRO C. BRIBRIESCO, MD
Staff Surgeon, Department of Thoracic
Surgery, Thoracic and Cardiovascular Surgery
Institute, Cleveland Clinic Foundation,
Cleveland, Ohio

CONNOR J. BRIDGES, BS
The Geisel School of Medicine at Dartmouth,
Hanover, New Hampshire

STEPHANIE H. CHANG, MD, MSCI
Associate Professor, Division of Thoracic
Surgery, Department of Cardiothoracic
Surgery, New York University Langone Health,
New York, New York

NICOLAS CONTRERAS, MD
Cardiothoracic Surgeon, Division of
Cardiothoracic Surgery, Department of
Surgery, University of Utah Health, Huntsman
Cancer Institute, Salt Lake City, Utah

MARTA ENGELKING, MD
Resident, Division of Thoracic and Foregut
Surgery, Department of General Surgery,
University of Minnesota, Minneapolis,
Minnesota

TRAVIS C. GERACI, MD
Assistant Professor, Division of Thoracic
Surgery, Department of Cardiothoracic
Surgery, New York University Langone Health,
New York, New York

DEVIN GILLASPIE, MD
Assistant Professor, Division of Acute Care
Surgery, Department of Surgery, University of
Tennessee Medical Center, Knoxville,
Tennessee

ERIN A. GILLASPIE, MD, MPH, FACS
Associate Professor with Tenure, Chief,
Division of Thoracic Surgery, Creighton
University Medical Center CHI Health, Omaha,
Nebraska

LAWRENCE E. GREITEN, MD, MSc
Associate Professor of Pediatric
Cardiothoracic Surgery, Department of
Surgery, University of Arkansas for Medical
Sciences, Arkansas Children's Hospital, Little
Rock, Arkansas

RIAN M. HASSON, MD, MPH
Surgeon, Department of Surgery, Section of
Thoracic Surgery, Dartmouth-Hitchcock
Medical Center, Lebanon, New Hampshire;

Geisel School of Medicine at Dartmouth, Hanover, New Hampshire; The Dartmouth Institute of Health Policy and Clinical Practice, Lebanon, New Hampshire

DOUGLAS Z. LIOU, MD
Clinical Associate Professor, Division of Thoracic Surgery, Department of Cardiothoracic Surgery, Stanford School of Medicine, Stanford, California

NATALIE S. LUI, MD
Assistant Professor, Division of Thoracic Surgery, Department of Cardiothoracic Surgery, Stanford School of Medicine, Stanford, California

BRIAN MITZMAN, MD, MS
Assistant Professor, Division of Cardiothoracic Surgery, Department of Surgery, University of Utah Health, Huntsman Cancer Institute, Salt Lake City, Utah

DINA AL RAMENI, MD
Resident/Fellow, Division of Cardiothoracic Surgery, Department of Surgery, University of Arizona - College of Medicine, Tucson, Arizona

RYAN J. RANDLE, MD
Resident Physician, Department of Surgery, Oregon Health and Science University, Portland, Oregon; Division of Thoracic Surgery, Department of Cardiothoracic Surgery, Stanford School of Medicine, Stanford, California

MADHURI RAO, MD
Assistant Professor, Division of Thoracic and Foregut Surgery, University of Minnesota, Minneapolis, Minnesota

MONISHA SUDARSHAN, MD, MPH
Staff Surgeon, Department of Thoracic Surgery, Thoracic and Cardiovascular Surgery Institute, Cleveland Clinic Foundation, Cleveland, Ohio

SADIA TASNIM, MD
Resident Physician, Department of General Surgery, Digestive Disease Institute, Thoracic and Cardiovascular Surgery Institute, Cleveland Clinic Foundation, Cleveland, Ohio

ROBERT J. VANDEWALLE, MD, MBA
Assistant Professor of Pediatric General Surgery, Pediatric Surgical Critical Care, Department of Surgery, University of Arkansas for Medical Sciences, Arkansas Children's Hospital, Little Rock, Arkansas

THOMAS K. VARGHESE Jr, MD, MS, MBA
Associate Chief Medical Quality Officer, Division of Cardiothoracic Surgery, Department of Surgery, University of Utah Health, Huntsman Cancer Institute, Salt Lake City, Utah

STEPHANIE G. WORRELL, MD
Associate Professor, Division of Cardiothoracic Surgery, Department of Surgery, University of Arizona - College of Medicine, Section Chief Thoracic Surgery, University of Arizona, Tucson, Arizona

CAMILLE YONGUE, MD
Cardiothoracic Surgery Resident, Division of Thoracic Surgery, Department of Cardiothoracic Surgery, New York University Langone Health, New York, New York

Contents

symptomatic patients with an elevated diaphragm. Plication can be approached either from a thoracic or abdominal approach, though most thoracic surgeons perform minimally invasive thoracoscopic plication. The goal of plication is to improve lung volumes and decrease paradoxic elevation of the hemidiaphragm. Diaphragm plication is safe, has excellent outcomes, and is associated with symptom improvement.

Management of Diaphragm Tumors   189
Marta Engelking and Madhuri Rao

Diaphragm tumors are very rare, with secondary tumors being more common than primary tumors. The most common benign primary tumors include lipomas and cysts, and malignant primary tumors include rhabdomyosarcoma and leiomyosarcoma. Endometriosis is the most common benign secondary tumor, followed by malignant tumors with localized spread of disease. In addition, widely metastatic disease has been described. Benign lipomas and cysts can be managed conservatively, but more complex or concerning disease typically requires resection. The diaphragm can often be repaired primarily, though any large defect or tension would indicate the need for mesh or an autologous reconstruction.

THORACIC SURGERY CLINICS

SERIES OF RELATED INTEREST

Advances in Surgery
http://www.advancessurgery.com/

Surgical Clinics
http://www.surgical.theclinics.com/

Surgical Oncology Clinics
https://www.surgonc.theclinics.com/

THE CLINICS ARE AVAILABLE ONLINE!
Access your subscription at:
www.theclinics.com

Foreword
To Eat and To Breathe, Respect the Diaphragm

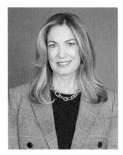

Virginia R. Litle, MD
Consulting Editor

As general thoracic surgeons, we primarily focus on lung cancer, esophageal disease, and mediastinal lesions. The diaphragm is sort of the stepchild of intrathoracic pathology. Fortunately, our invited guest editor for this issue of *Thoracic Surgery Clinics* entitled "Surgical Conditions of the Diaphragm" has taken a special interest in this organ. Guest Editor Dr Erin Gillaspie has shared her succinctly detailed technical videos of robotic diaphragm plication at our meetings, so she was an obvious expert to invite to edit this issue. Thank you to Dr Gillaspie for identifying and inviting a diversity of authors (including her trauma surgeon sister!).

Starting off with Dr Monisha Sudarshan and Cleveland Clinic colleagues, we are reminded of how we should respect the diaphragm given its key role in respiration and gastrointestinal function. They include fun facts that take us back to med school and surgery training—diaphragmatic anatomy and physiology. Some reminders include (1) 50% of our work of breathing originates from the diaphragm muscles, and for marathoners, that

would be at least 80%; (2) Avoid radial incisions to preserve phrenic branches, and when doing the safest incision—circumferential—mark with sutures to assist with realignment when closing; and (3) Morgagni hernias are more common in women and obese patients, who typically present with right substernal pain. For those thoracic surgeons at trauma facilities encountering a penetrating injury below T4, think possible diaphragm injury. Beyond respiratory function and in the hernia category, the diaphragm is also integral to the management of foregut disease—reflux, emesis, and competency of the lower esophageal sphincter. Two integral roles of diaphragm physiology to survival—breathing and eating.

Drs Maddy Rao and Marta Engelking provide a nice synopsis of the rare tumors of the diaphragm. We probably don't think of catamenial pneumothoraces as tumor cases, but endometriosis is considered a benign tumor—and it can involve the diaphragm. So can schwannomas, leiomyomas, and other fascinomas. A take-home message is the reminder that autologous tissue can

Thorac Surg Clin 34 (2024) ix–x
https://doi.org/10.1016/j.thorsurg.2024.02.003
1547-4127/24/© 2024 Elsevier Inc. All rights reserved.

thoracic.theclinics.com

be used to close diaphragmatic defects, such as serratus, rectus, and the latissimus. Drs Stephanie Worrell and Rameni expand on the topic of reconstructive techniques for diaphragm resection in their contribution and list several synthetic meshes that would be useful as well as bioprosthetic meshes for contaminated fields.

Thank you to Dr Gillaspie and to *all* the contributors to this issue, a detailed compendium of diaphragm management. Don't let the diaphragm be put on the irrelevant back burner. Remember it's C3, 4, and 5 that keep us alive!

Take a big breath and enjoy reading this quarterly monograph.

Virginia R. Litle, MD
St. Elizabeth's Medical Center
11 Nevins Street, Suite 201
Brighton, MA 02135, USA

E-mail address:
Vlitle@gmail.com

Twitter: @vlitlemd (V.R. Litle)

Preface
Delving into the Diaphragm

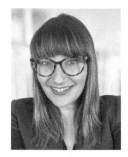

Erin A. Gillaspie, MD, MPH
Editor

The diaphragm serves many purposes in the body. While classically, the diaphragm is thought of as a critical muscle of respiration, and it is, the diaphragm serves a plethora of functions. This musculotendinous structure with its unique dome shape serves as an anatomic barrier between the abdomen and the chest, aids in the flow of blood and lymph, and even assists in the function of our gastrointestinal (GI) and genitourinary systems. Therefore, when the diaphragm sustains a traumatic injury, neurologic dysfunction, or diseases such as cancer or hernias, the impacts can manifest throughout the body.

Symptoms of diaphragm dysfunction vary dramatically, most commonly manifesting with GI or respiratory symptoms. In most cases, symptoms are mild, but some cases can progress to respiratory failure. Due to the rarity of diaphragm disorders and the subtlety of clinical presentation, many patients are misdiagnosed or have delayed diagnosis, which can impact quality of life and survival.

This issue of *Thoracic Surgery Clinics* titled "Surgical Conditions of the Diaphragm" focuses on all aspects of this important muscle. We open with three articles to help set the basis of care: morphologic structure and function, an article highlighting practical radiologic considerations, and round out with a summary of surgical considerations for approaching the diaphragm.

These three articles help to set the foundation for the rest of the issue that tackles specific diagnoses, recommended workup, tips and tricks on the surgical approach, and review of data on long-term outcomes. The topics covered include the management of congenital hernias both in infants and in adults, acquired diaphragmatic hernias, eventration and paralysis, primary and secondary cancers of the diaphragm, and unique considerations for traumatic injuries.

I am incredibly grateful for the extraordinary contributions of the authors and hope this comprehensive guide serves as an important tool in your practice to help with the management of diaphragm pathologies.

DISCLOSURES

Dr E.A. Gillaspie discloses the following: serves as speaker for BMS; and serves on the editorial board for BMS, AZ, and Genentech. None of the conflicts of interest are pertinent to this publication.

Erin A. Gillaspie, MD, MPH
Creighton University Medical Center CHI Health
7500 Mercy Road
Omaha, NE, USA

E-mail address:
eringillaspie@creighton.edu

Thorac Surg Clin 34 (2024) xi
https://doi.org/10.1016/j.thorsurg.2024.02.001
1547-4127/24/© 2024 Published by Elsevier Inc.

Surgical Diaphragm
Anatomy and Physiology

Sadia Tasnim, MD[a,b], Alejandro C. Bribriesco, MD[b], Monisha Sudarshan, MD, MPH[b],*

KEYWORDS

• Diaphragm • Anatomy • Physiology • Diaphragmatic hernia • Congenital hernia

KEY POINTS

- The diaphragm is a muscular aponeurotic structure composed of a central tendon and three muscular components, namely, pars lumbaris, pars costalis, and pars sternalis.
- The pars costalis plays a role in respiration and pars lumbaris in regulating gastrointestinal functions such as swallowing and emesis.
- Congenital diaphragmatic hernias occur from the failure of proper fusion of embryonic components.
- Hiatal hernias are the most common hernias resulting from a weakness or defect in the phrenoesophageal ligament.

INTRODUCTION

The diaphragm is a musculoaponeurotic structure that acts as a boundary between the thoracic and abdominal cavities. It serves a dual function in both respiration and maintaining gastrointestinal function. It is important for surgeons to understand the basic anatomy and physiology of the diaphragm as it is encountered in almost all thoracic surgery procedures. This article summarizes the anatomy and physiology of the diaphragm and its relevance to surgical procedures.

EMBRYOLOGY

The diaphragm is formed from the union of the septum transversum and the pleuroperitoneal folds (**Fig. 1**). The dorsal mesentery and the muscular body wall also contribute to the final structure of the diaphragm.[1,2] Septum transversum is derived from the embryonic mesoderm and contributes to the ventral portion of the diaphragm, in particular, the central tendon of the diaphragm. It separates the pericardium from the rest of the thorax and makes a trileaflet central tendon.

The leaflets are located in the right and left hemidiaphragm and underneath the pericardium.

The pleuroperitoneal folds make the dorsolateral portion of the diaphragm. Myotomes from C3, C4, and C5 migrate down the lateral border of the thorax to the center in the seventh week of life to form the central muscular component of the diaphragm. The lateral muscles of the diaphragm originate from myotomes carrying nerve innervations from T7 to T12. The diaphragm is formed starting from the third week of life and completed before the return of the intestines into the abdomen at the 10th week of life to prevent the migration of intestines to the chest. Improper formation of the diaphragm leads to congenital diaphragmatic hernia.[3] Finally, the dorsal mesentery of the esophagus attaches the foregut to the dorsal body wall which then develops into the diaphragmatic crura.

ANATOMY
Structure

Each hemidiaphragm is convex to the thoracic cavity and concave to the abdominal cavity.[4] The

[a] Department of General Surgery, Digestive Disease Institute, Cleveland Clinic Foundation, 9500 Euclid Avenue, Cleveland, OH 44195, USA; [b] Department of Thoracic Surgery, Thoracic and Cardiovascular Surgery Institute, Cleveland Clinic Foundation, 9500 Euclid Avenue, Cleveland, OH 44195, USA
* Corresponding author.
E-mail address: sudarsm2@ccf.org
Twitter: @_SadiaTasnim (S.T.); @abribriesco43 (A.C.B.); @Monisha_Sud_MD (M.S.)

Thorac Surg Clin 34 (2024) 111–118
https://doi.org/10.1016/j.thorsurg.2024.01.002

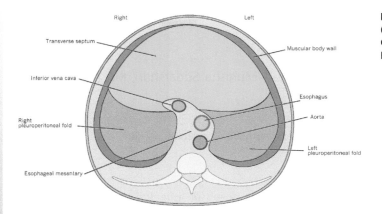

Fig. 1. Embryology of the diaphragm. (*Reprinted with permission,* Cleveland Clinic Foundation ©2023. All Rights Reserved.)

concavity allows abdominal organs such as the liver and spleen to be protected by the lower ribs cage. The diaphragm has two main structural components: the central tendon and the muscular portion (**Box 1**). **Fig. 2** shows the structures of the diaphragm from the thoracic cavity, and **Fig. 3** shows the structures of the diaphragm from the abdominal cavity.

Central tendon
The central tendon is a noncontractile aponeurotic band with three leaflets.[5] The right leaflet is the largest leaflet. Unlike its name, the central tendon is located more anteriorly and underneath the pericardium.

Muscular portion
These striated skeletal muscle fibers originate ventral to the psoas and quadratus lumborum muscle from the aponeurotic arch of the ligamentum arcuatum externum. There are three muscular parts.

Crural/lumbar part (pars lumbaris) This is the strongest portion of the diaphragm and has a muscular and tendinous component. The right crus originates from the L3–4 and the left crus from the L1–2 vertebral bodies. The right crus is larger and longer than the left. The right crus splits to form the esophageal hiatus in more than 60% of individuals.[5,6] The remaining 40% is formed by the contribution of both the right and left crus. The tendon provides the strength to secure sutures during a cruroplasty. The right crus also forms the ligament of Treitz.

Costal part (pars costalis) The costal part of the diaphragm is formed by muscle fibers originating from the posterior surface of ribs 5–10 radiating to the central tendon.

Sternal part (pars sternalis) The sternal part of the diaphragm is formed by muscle fibers originating from the posterior surface of the xiphoid process which then joins the central tendon.

Pleural and peritoneal attachments
The pleura attaches to the convex surface on the thoracic side of the diaphragm. It can be difficult to distinguish the pleura and the central tendon of the diaphragm due to the similarity of color and texture of the two structures. There is a diaphragmatic recess of about 1 cm diameter that does not contain pleura. This recess is used during the extrapleural dissection to facilitate exposure of the muscles of diaphragm for division. The peritoneum covers the concave surface or abdominal side of the diaphragm.

Blood Supply

Arteries
The diaphragm is supplied by the superior and inferior phrenic, musculophrenic, pericardiophrenic, and intercostal arteries. The superior phrenic arteries reside on the thoracic side of the diaphragm and originate from the thoracic aorta. They supply the thoracic side of the diaphragm (see **Fig. 2**). The inferior phrenic arteries are on the abdominal side of the diaphragm and typically originating from either the aorta or the celiac artery or the renal arteries. The right inferior phrenic passes behind the vena cava, whereas the left inferior phrenic artery passes posterior to the esophagus and then runs anteriorly along the lateral side of the esophageal hiatus (see **Fig. 3**). The left and right inferior phrenic arteries divide into the medial and lateral branches. The medial branches collateralize to the musculophrenic and pericardiophrenic arteries. The lateral branches collateralize to the intercostal arteries.

- The diaphragm is a muscular aponeurotic structure composed of a central tendon and three muscular components, namely, pars lumbaris, pars costalis, and pars sternalis.
- The diaphragm is supplied by the superior and inferior phrenic arteries, musculophrenic and pericardiophrenic arteries, and intercostal arteries. Veins follow the path of the arteries.
- The diaphragm is innervated by the right and left phrenic nerves whose nerve roots originate from C3, C4, and C5 along with the sixth and seventh intercostal nerves.

The musculophrenic and pericardiophrenic arteries originate from the internal thoracic arteries after they pass through the foramen of Morgagni and Larrey on the right and left side, respectively. The internal thoracic arteries then continue distally as the superior epigastric arteries. The musculophrenic and pericardiophrenic arteries also supply the phrenic nerves and pericardial fat.[7] Finally, the peripheral costal diaphragm is supplied by the intercostal arteries.

Diaphragmatic blood flow is contingent on the mechanism of breathing. A balance between the intra-abdominal and intramuscular pressure regulates the blood flow to the diaphragm. At rest, with diaphragmatic relaxation, the blood flow increases and during inspiration it decreases—particularly with forced inspiration due to increased intramuscular pressure as the diaphragm contracts.[8]

Veins

The venous anatomy of the diaphragm parallels the arteries. The superior phrenic veins drain into the internal thoracic veins. The right inferior phrenic vein drains into the inferior vena cava. One branch of the left inferior phrenic vein drains to the left renal or suprarenal vein; the other passes anterior to the esophageal hiatus and empties into the vena cava.

Innervation

The diaphragm is innervated by the right and left phrenic nerves whose nerve roots originate from C3, C4, and C5 along with sixth and seventh intercostal nerves. The phrenic nerves run craniocaudally, passing anterior to the lung hilum and divide at the level of the diaphragm. The right phrenic enters the diaphragm lateral to the inferior vena cava, and the left phrenic enters lateral to the heart. Each phrenic nerve splits into an anterior and posterior trunk. The anterior trunk divides into the sternal and the anterolateral branch. The posterior trunk divides into the crural and posterolateral branch (see **Figs. 2** and **3**). The two lateral branches are significantly longer than the sternal and crural branches and innervate most of the diaphragm. The right phrenic is rarely medial to the internal thoracic artery, whereas the left phrenic is mostly medial to left internal thoracic artery, making the left nerve prone to injuries during harvest of the left internal thoracic artery for bypass.[9] The position of the right and left phrenic nerves is also important to consider during minimally invasive thymectomy.

Diaphragmatic Incisions

Incision on the diaphragm should be planned carefully to avoid excessive bleeding and denervation, leading to the weakness and hemiparesis of the diaphragm. Four types of incisions are discussed: (A) radial, (B) circumferential, (C) transverse radial, and (D) linear (**Fig. 4**). Radial incisions from the

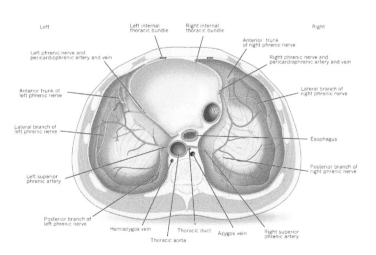

Fig. 2. Superior view of the diaphragm (*Reprinted with permission*, Cleveland Clinic Foundation ©2023. All Rights Reserved.).

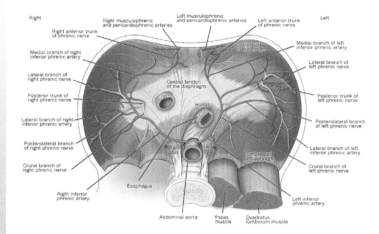

Fig. 3. Inferior view of the diaphragm (*Reprinted with permission*, Cleveland Clinic Foundation ©2023. All Rights Reserved.)

costal margin to the esophageal hiatus (A) can cause serious injury to the crural and posterolateral branches of the phrenic nerves, and therefore, this incision is rarely performed. A circumferential (B) incision is performed 2 to 3 cm inward from the costal margin and 5 cm lateral to the edge of the central tendon to avoid the antero- and posterolateral branches of the phrenic nerves. It is considered to be the safest incision, however, can become difficult to align during closure. Placing marking sutures or clips helps to ensure careful realignment of the diaphragm during closure. This incision is usually used in a thoracoabdominal approach. Some of the less common incisions are the transverse radial and linear incision. Transverse radial incisions (C) are safer than radial as they course between the branches of the phrenic nerves. Finally, linear incisions avoiding the nerve branches are another alternative (**Box 2**).

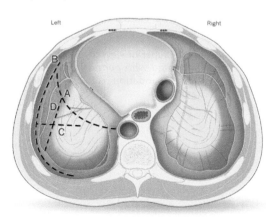

Fig. 4. Diaphragmatic incisions. A. Radial. B. Circumferential. C. Transverse radial. D. Linear. (*Reprinted with permission*, Cleveland Clinic Foundation ©2023. All Rights Reserved.)

Lymphatics

Anteriorly the diaphragmatic lymphatic chain drains to the parasternal nodes and ultimately the internal thoracic chain. Posteriorly, they drain into the brachiocephalic and parasternal nodes and ultimately to the thoracic duct. Disruption of these lymphatic chains during surgical procedures can result in chylothorax of chylous ascites.

Major Diaphragmatic Openings

The diaphragm has three major openings allowing inferior vena cava, esophagus, and aorta to pass from the thoracic cavity to the abdominal cavity.

Vena cava opening
The vena cava opening is at the level of T8 in the right hemithorax. This is the most anterior of the formal diaphragmatic openings allowing the vena cava and the right phrenic nerve to pass through.

Box 2
Surgical considerations
• To avoid injury to the phrenic nerve, a circumferential incision is the least traumatizing and safest but requires careful planning and marking for proper alignment during closure.
• The tendon of the crus holds the sutures during the cruroplasty of a hiatal hernia repair.
• Acute diaphragmatic injuries are assessed most commonly via laparoscopy or laparotomy. They may also be assessed via thoracoscopy or thoracotomy. Delayed presentation of a diaphragm injury may require transthoracic approach secondary to the potential development of adhesion between thoracic structures and herniated abdominal contents.

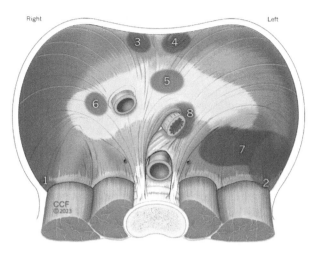

Right   Left

CCF
©2023

Fig. 5. Diaphragmatic openings and weaknesses. 1. Right lumbosacral triangle. 2. Left lumbosacral triangle. 3. Foramen of Morgagni. 4. Foramen of Larrey. 5. Peritoneopericardial communication (septum transversum defect). 6. Paracaval hernia. 7. Pleuroperitoneal hernia. 8. Hiatal hernia. (*Reprinted with permission*, Cleveland Clinic Foundation ©2023. All Rights Reserved.)

Esophageal opening

The esophageal opening is at the level of T10 located slightly left of the midline. The aperture is anteriorly bordered by the right crus and posteriorly by the median arcuate ligament. The esophagus, anterior and posterior vagal trunks, phrenicoabdominal (sensory) branch of the left phrenic nerve, esophageal branch of left gastric artery, and vein pass through this opening.

Aortic opening

The aortic opening is at the level of T12 located in the left hemithorax. This is the most posterior opening bordered posteriorly by the vertebral body, laterally by the crura and anteriorly by the median arcuate ligaments. The aorta, azygous, and hemi azygous veins, aortic plexus and lymphatic vessels, and thoracic duct pass through this opening.

Minor Diaphragmatic Openings and Weaknesses

Apart from the major openings of the diaphragm, there are some minor openings or congenital weaknesses that can be potential spaces for organ herniation. The more common of them are discussed as follows.

a. Foramen of Bochdalek: The foramen of Bochdalek is located at the lumbosacral triangle between the lumbar and costal part of the diaphragm bilaterally (**Fig. 5**: 1 and 2).
b. Foramen of Morgagni and Larrey: The foramen of Morgagni is a triangular potential space in the right parasternal area (see **Fig. 5**: 3). The foramen of Larrey is in the left parasternal area (see **Fig. 5**: 4). The internal thoracic vessels pass through these foramens.

c. Others: Other less commonly known minor weaknesses of the diaphragm are the peritoneopericardial (see **Fig. 5**: 5), paracaval (see **Fig. 5**: 6), and pleuroperitoneal foramens (see **Fig. 5**: 7).

Congenital diaphragmatic hernias

The failure of fusion of the pleuroperitoneal membrane with the septum transversum or the muscular body wall can lead to actual defects or congenital hernias.

a. Bochdalek hernia: Bochdalek hernias are the most common congenital diaphragmatic hernias accounting for 95% of these hernias.[3] They occur primarily in the left posterior hemidiaphragm.
b. Morgagni hernia: Accounting for only 3% of congenital hernias requiring surgical repair.[10] The most common presenting symptom for Morgagni hernias is right-sided substernal pain. These hernias are more common in women and obese patients.[11] The foramen of Larrey is covered by the pericardial sac, so herniation is less common through this foramen.
c. Right-sided congenital diaphragmatic hernia: Commonly seen in children due to failure of the septum transversum and pleuroperitoneal membranes to close.

Traumatic diaphragmatic hernia

Traumatic diaphragmatic injuries can be blunt or penetrating. Any penetrating injury at or below the T4 level increases concern for a diaphragmatic injury. On the other hand, blunt injuries increase intra-abdominal pressure causing rupture of the diaphragm, usually seen as a seat belt injury in a motor vehicle accident. The left side is more susceptible than the right due to the protective nature of the liver on the right side. Acute diaphragmatic injuries are explored via laparoscopy or laparotomy with potential need to place a chest tube to prevent tension pneumothorax during insufflation.

Hiatal hernia

The most common diaphragmatic hernia is a hiatal hernia.[12] There are four types of hiatal hernias: Types I–IV. Type I or sliding hiatal hernia is the most common accounting for 90% to 95% of hiatal hernias. This involves the weakening of the phrenoesophageal ligament and displacement of the gastroesophageal junction into the chest (see **Fig. 5**: 8). The most common presenting symptom for these hernias is reflux. Types II–IV are also called paraesophageal hernias due to herniation of fundus of the gastroesophageal junction, stomach, or other organs into the chest. Type II also involves the weakening of the phrenoesophageal ligament and displacement of only the gastric fundus into the chest keeping the gastroesophageal junction and cardia in the abdomen. Type III is a combination of Type I and Type II where both the gastric fundus and gastroesophageal junction are in the chest. Finally, Type IV involves the herniation of another organ such as colon or spleen or pancreas in the chest.

These hernias are associated with large defects in the phrenoesophageal membrane and widening of the hiatus. As time progresses the hernia enlarges and the positive pressure in abdomen pushes the abdominal organs toward the negative pressure in the thorax. A special group of these paraesophageal hernias are the giant paraesophageal hernias, defined as greater than two-third of stomach in chest. These hernias have a propensity to volvulize along the short or long axis. Volvulus along the long axis known as organo-axial volvulus is more common than volvulus along the short axis known as mesentero-axial volvulus.

PHYSIOLOGY

Apart from providing anatomic stability and separating the thoracic and abdominal organs, the diaphragm has two main functions: respiration and assistance in gastrointestinal function (**Box 3**).

Role in Respiration

The diaphragm is the most important respiratory muscle followed by the intercostal and scalene muscles. The costal portion of the diaphragm assists in respiration. At rest, the central tendon is displaced toward the chest due to positive intra-abdominal pressure. The right hemidiaphragm lies at the level of fourth intercostal space and the left hemidiaphragm at the level of the fifth intercostal

---

Box 3
Physiology

- Pars costalis plays a role in respiration and pars lumbaris in regulating gastrointestinal functions.
- The diaphragm displaces two rib spaces to initiate negative intrathoracic pressure for inspiration.
- The crura relax to allow food boluses to enter and contracts to prevent reflux.

---

space. During inspiration, the radial muscle fibers contract pulling the diaphragm down and flat. The central tendon is moved about two rib spaces caudally. The first rib is elevated and fixed by the scalene muscles of the neck. The lower ribs are raised by the external intercostal muscles. The coordination of these actions creates a negative pressure in the thoracic cavity and allows for atmospheric air to be drawn into the lungs. In contrast, expiration is passive and occurs by the elastic recoil of the relaxing muscles, as the diaphragm returns to the resting position.

Diaphragmatic dysfunction ranges from an inability to generate sufficient pressure (weakness) to complete loss of function (paralysis).[13] These can be secondary to age, neuromuscular or inflammatory disease processes, trauma, surgery, mechanical ventilation, and so forth. Chest x-ray is the most readily available test. Ultrasound of the diaphragm is becoming more popular and used at high-volume centers (**Fig. 6**). Normally functioning diaphragm shows excursion of the diaphragm in a tidal breathing pattern. This image is best acquired from the anterior axillary window using a phased array probe at the 7th to 8th intercostal space (see **Fig. 6** I). A completely paralyzed diaphragm may show no movement (**Fig. 6** II) or paradoxic motion (see **Fig. 6** III) on ultrasound. Finally using a linear probe at the 7th to 8th intercostal space, thickening can be observed when the diaphragm transitions from a point of relaxation (A) to contraction (B) (see **Fig. 6** IV).

Each hemidiaphragm contributes to about 25% of the work of breathing and the remaining is supplied by intercostal muscles. During exertion, the diaphragm can increase its workload to 80%.[14] Another important clinical consideration is diaphragmatic muscle atrophy from prolonged mechanical ventilation resulting in difficulty weaning from the ventilator.[15]

Role in Gastrointestinal Functions

A commonly overlooked function of the diaphragm is the role it plays in the gastrointestinal function. The

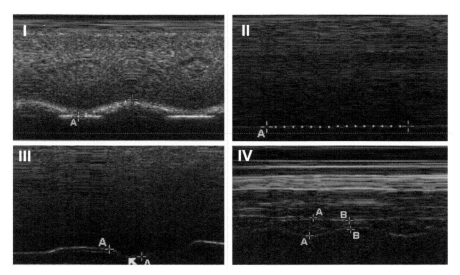

Fig. 6. Ultrasonography of the diaphragm. (I) Normal: The hyperechoic line represents the excursion of the diaphragm in a tidal breathing pattern. (II) Paralyzed or dysfunctional diaphragm (no movement). (III) Paralyzed or dysfunctional diaphragm (paradoxic movement). When a Sniff maneuver is performed, there is a paradoxic motion as demonstrated at the point of downward deflection of the hyperechoic line (A). (IV) Diaphragmatic thickening: Using a linear probe at the 7th to 8th intercostal space, thickening can be observed when the diaphragm transitions from a point of relaxation (A) to contraction (B). (*Courtesy of* Dr. Jason Dean, MSN, APRN, FNP-C from the Respiratory Institute of the Cleveland Clinic Foundation.)

crural part of the diaphragm assists in esophageal emptying, reflux barrier, and emesis. As a food bolus enters the esophagus, the crura relax to let food pass and contract acting as a reflux barrier afterward. Emesis is a complex mechanism where the diaphragm and the abdominal muscles coordinate to expel gastric content. The contraction of the costal part of the diaphragm and the abdominal muscles increases intra-abdominal pressure, whereas the crural part of the diaphragm relaxes to allow food to come back up through the esophagus.[16]

SUMMARY

The diaphragm is a complex anatomic structure supporting both respiratory and gastrointestinal function. Surgery of the diaphragm requires a thoughtful understanding of the anatomic relationships, to optimize outcome while maintaining function.

CLINICS CARE POINTS

- The right crus splits to form the esophageal hiatus in more than 60% of individuals (whereas in the rest, the esophageal crura is derived by the contribution of both crura).
- The tendon of the crus holds the sutures during the reconstruction of the hiatus.

- A circumferential incision of the diaphragm is the least traumatizing and safest but requires careful planning and marking for proper alignment during closure.

ACKNOWLEDGMENTS

The authors would like to thank Jason Dean, MSN, APRN, FNP-C from the Respiratory Institute of the Cleveland Clinic Foundation for providing the ultrasound images of the diaphragm.

DISCLOSURE

The authors have nothing to disclose.

REFERENCES

1. De Leon N, Tse WH, Ameis D, et al. Embryology and anatomy of congenital diaphragmatic hernia. Semin Pediatr Surg 2022;31(6):151229.
2. Schumpelick V, Steinau G, Schlüper I, et al. Surgical embryology and anatomy of the diaphragm with surgical applications. Surg Clin North Am 2000;80(1):213–39.
3. Robinson PD, Fitzgerald DA. Congenital diaphragmatic hernia. Paediatr Respir Rev 2007;8(4):323–34.
4. Bains KNS, Kashyap S, Lappin SL. Anatomy, thorax, diaphragm. Available at:. In: StatPearls. StatPearls

Publishing; 2023 http://www.ncbi.nlm.nih.gov/books/NBK519558/. [Accessed 1 July 2023].

5. Baaj AA, Papadimitriou K, Amin AG, et al. Surgical anatomy of the diaphragm in the anterolateral approach to the spine: a cadaveric study. J Spinal Disord Tech 2014;27(4):220.

6. Collis JL, Kelly TD, Wiley AM. Anatomy of the crura of the diaphragm and the surgery of hiatus hernia. Thorax 1954;9(3):175–89.

7. Anderson TM, Miller JI. Surgical technique and application of pericardial fat pad and pericardiophrenic grafts. Ann Thorac Surg 1995;59(6):1590–1.

8. Supinski GS, DiMarco AF, Altose MD. Effect of diaphragmatic contraction on intramuscular pressure and vascular impedance. J Appl Physiol Bethesda Md 1985 1990;68(4):1486–93.

9. Owens WA, Gladstone DJ, Heylings DJ. Surgical anatomy of the phrenic nerve and internal mammary artery. Ann Thorac Surg 1994;58(3):843–4.

10. Hussong RL, Landreneau RJ, Cole FH. Diagnosis and repair of a Morgagni hernia with video-assisted thoracic surgery. Ann Thorac Surg 1997;63(5):1474–5.

11. Adereti C, Zahir J, Robinson E, et al. A case report and literature review on incidental Morgagni hernia in bariatric patients: to repair or not to repair? Cureus 2023;15(6):e39950.

12. Smith RE, Shahjehan RD. Hiatal hernia. Available at:. In: StatPearls. StatPearls Publishing; 2023 http://www.ncbi.nlm.nih.gov/books/NBK562200/. [Accessed 25 July 2023].

13. McCool FD, Tzelepis GE. Dysfunction of the diaphragm. N Engl J Med 2012;366(10):932–42.

14. Wade OL. Movements of the thoracic cage and diaphragm in respiration. J Physiol 1954;124(2):193–212.

15. Levine S, Nguyen T, Taylor N, et al. Rapid disuse atrophy of diaphragm fibers in mechanically ventilated humans. N Engl J Med 2008;358(13):1327–35.

16. Delattre JF, Palot JP, Ducasse A, et al. The crura of the diaphragm and diaphragmatic passage. Applications to gastroesophageal reflux, its investigation and treatment. Anat Clin 1985;7(4):271–83.

Imaging of the Diaphragm
A Primer

Erin A. Gillaspie, MD, MPH

KEYWORDS

• MRI • Computed tomography scan • Fluoroscopy • Ultrasound • Diaphragm

KEY POINTS

- There are multiple imaging modalities that may be used to evaluate the diaphragm. Each has a unique indication, benefits, and drawbacks.
- Chest X ray is the most common imaging modality of the chest. This is often coupled with a secondary image to help further delineate pathology.
- Ultrasound is a radiation-free technique that can provide rapid interpretation and both morphologic and functional data.
- A sniff test, the fluoroscopic assessment of the diaphragm, has long stood as the gold standard for the diagnosis of diaphragmatic paralysis.
- Computed tomography scan and MRI technology provide a wide field of view, 3-dimensional presentation, and a comprehensive morphologic assessment of the diaphragm.

INTRODUCTION

The diaphragm is a dome-shaped musculotendinous structure that provides a physical separation of the thorax from the abdomen and plays a critical role in respiratory function. It also plays a minor role in the gastrointestinal and urinary systems.

Disorders of the diaphragm which are discussed in detail within the sections of this article include traumatic, oncologic, neurogenic, and anatomic abnormalities such as congenital and acquired hernias. Any kind of perturbation of normal function from the aforementioned abnormalities may lead to diaphragm dysfunction and respiratory impairment.

Patients may present with a variety of symptoms ranging from asymptomatic to cough, pain, nausea, dysphagia, dyspnea or even an inability to perform activities of daily living.

Due to the rarity of diaphragm disorders, they are often overlooked or misdiagnosed. Radiography plays a critical role in the assessment of patients with diaphragmatic pathology and the considerations for each modality are discussed herein.

IMAGING MODALITIES

There are many imaging options to consider for the assessment of the diaphragm and selection should be made based on the information required for diagnosis and to help guide therapy. Chest X ray (CXR) and computed tomography (CT), for example, are static techniques that are excellent for morphologic or anatomic assessment of the diaphragm but less useful for assessing function.[1] Fluoroscopy, ultrasound, and MRI are dynamic imaging modalities that can provide morphologic and functional assessment of the diaphragm.[1-3]

Chest X Ray

Plain film imaging remains the most common diagnostic radiographic modality used. The technology leverages electromagnetic radiation, focused on a particular anatomic region, and once the radiation passes through the patient, a receptor captures photons ultimately forming an image. Despite the ease and availability of plain films, they are limited by challenges of dimensionality, overlying structures that may obscure the anatomy of interest, or patient factors such as limited inspiration.[4]

Division of Thoracic Surgery, Creighton University Medical Center, 7500 Mercy Boulevard, Omaha, NE 68124, USA
E-mail address: erin.gillaspie@commonspirit.org

Thorac Surg Clin 34 (2024) 119–125
https://doi.org/10.1016/j.thorsurg.2024.02.002

Initial assessment of the diaphragm is performed most commonly with CXR.[1] The study is readily available in most centers, cost effective, fast, and has low radiation exposure. The details can be enhanced by obtaining additional views. An anterior and posterior (**Fig. 1**A), and lateral (**Fig. 1**B) views are obtained most commonly but even decubitus views may be selected. The study can provide important morphologic information about the diaphragm including shape, relative position both compared to adjacent structures and the contralateral diaphragm, sharpness, and, in some cases, even defects.[2]

CXR is often coupled with other imaging modalities to afford greater assessment of anatomy or function of the diaphragm as interpretation can be challenging and signs are subtle or nonspecific. The following table summarizes some common plain imaging findings for diaphragmatic pathologies (**Table 1**).[5-7]

Ultrasound

Ultrasonography of the diaphragm dates back to the 1960s as a tool to determine the shape and motion of the diaphragm.[8] This modality gained popularity and in 1989, when Dr Wait and colleagues published their seminal paper on M mode ultrasonography to measure diaphragm thickness during the respiratory cycle creating a thickness fraction to help assess function.[9]

Ultrasound is a noninvasive technique, is portable, and has no radiation exposure. The technology leverages sound waves above audible ranges (20,000 Hz). The transducer (probes) contains a piezoelectric crystal that sends acoustic waves into the tissues. The propagation speed of the acoustic wave is determined by the stiffness of the tissues the wave travels through—fastest through solids and slowest through gas. Some of the sound waves are reflected back toward the probe (echo), some will be absorbed, and some scattered. Several million cycles of sending and listening for returning waves occur every second

and are ultimately converted into images on the monitor. The frequency selected should be determined by the location of the tissues. Lower frequency is able to penetrate deeper into tissue, but this compromises resolution. Brightness mode ultrasound (B mode) provides useful structural information with different shades of gray corresponding to returning amplitudes or echoes. Motion mode (M mode) captures movement of structures in 1 line of the B mode. These 2 modalities are often coupled. Doppler or color Doppler may be added to show blood or fluid flow through a structure.[10]

Diaphragmatic anatomy can be assessed on B mode ultrasound and reveals a 3-layered structure with 2 echogenic layers of pleura and a hypoechoic layer of muscle in between (**Fig. 2**). In M mode, the thickness of the diaphragm and movement of the diaphragm may be assessed. In a normal diaphragm, the diaphragm is thinnest at end exhalation and thickest during contraction at end inhalation—of note, forceful inhalation will create greater thickness than passive breathing.[8]

Generally, the diaphragm is assessed with a high-frequency linear probe in the anterior axillary line, between the 8th and 10th intercostal spaces.[8,11] The diaphragm is first assessed on B mode to help gather anatomic detail prior to adding M mode for dynamic assessment during respiration.[8] Curvilinear probes (lower frequency) can be useful in dynamic assessment. The probe is positioned between the anterior and mid-clavicular lines and oriented perpendicular to the dome of the liver on the right or the spleen on the left.[8] During passive respiratory, the diaphragm excursion varies by patient factors but is approximately 1 cm during quiet breathing, 1.6 to 1.8 cm during voluntary sniffing, and 3.7 to 4.7 cm during deep breathing.[12]

Ultrasound may be used to evaluate diaphragmatic motion and defects, and more recently, it has gained traction as an adjunctive assessment of intensive care unit patients to help determine readiness for extubation.[11,13]

Ultrasound, like CXR, does have some drawbacks including variability in image collection and

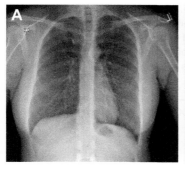
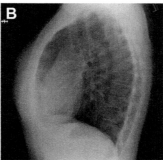

Fig. 1. Anterior and posterior (*A*) and lateral (*B*) chest radiographs. Note the domed, smooth shape of the diaphragms. The right diaphragm is slightly elevated when compared to the left, due to its cephalad displacement from the underlying liver. The costophrenic and cardiophrenic angles are sharp and there are no notable diaphragmatic defects. (*Courtesy of* Dr. Tom McLaren.)

Table 1
Common plain imaging findings for diaphragmatic pathologies

Diagnosis	Radiographic Features
Eventration	Upward bulging of the diaphragm on 1 side, most commonly involving the anterior most portion of the diaphragm. This may manifest as a double-density sign on the ipsilateral side. The elevation of the anterior portion of the diaphragm is best viewed on a lateral view film. The mediastinum may deviate towards the contralateral side to facilitate expansion of the ipsilateral lung that may be atelectatic.
Paralysis	Normally the right dome of the diaphragm is higher in position as compared to the left dome; if the left dome of the diaphragm is elevated (>2 cm), diaphragmatic palsy should be suspected.
Hernias	Symptomatic and asymptomatic defects may be identified on plain chest X ray manifesting with an air bubble above the diaphragm, often with some narrowing as the structure passes through the diaphragm. Fat-containing hernias such as a posterior Bochdalek may also be visualized, particularly on a lateral view as a rounded structure with increased density along the posterior chest wall.

From Verhey PT, Gosselin MV, Primack SL, Kraemer AC. Differentiating diaphragmatic paralysis and eventration. Acad Radiol. 2007;14 (4): 420-5. https://doi.org/10.1016/j.acra.2007.01.027; and Sandstrom CK, Stern EJ. Diaphragm hernias: a spectrum of radiographic appearances. Curr Prob Diag Radiol. 2011, 40(3):95-115.

interpretation. Even the measurement of diaphragm thickness is subject to observer disagreement secondary to the rib space through which the diaphragm is analyzed.[14] There is no question that

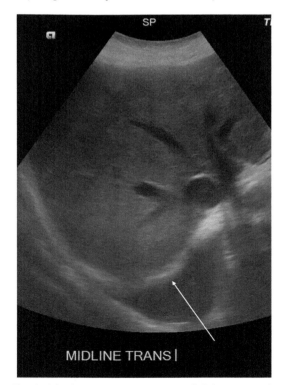

Fig. 2. Diaphragmatic anatomy on brightness mode ultrasound reveals 2 echogenic layers of the pleura sandwiching the hypoechoic muscle. (*Courtesy of* Dr. Tom McLaren.)

there are also limits to the field of view—both diaphragms cannot be easily visualized simultaneously, significantly domed diaphragm can be more difficult to assess as it traverses multiple rib spaces, and visibility can be limited by gaseous distention of abdominal viscera, pleural effusion, and other thoracic and abdominal pathologies.[3,15]

Fluoroscopy

The use of diagnostic fluoroscopy has been declining for decades, but remains a useful imaging modality, in particular for the diagnosis of diaphragm paralysis.[16,17] Fluoroscopy leverages similar techniques to a conventional plain film but rather than a single image, fluoroscopy captures 30+ images per second displaying dynamic processes such as respiration. The cumulative dose of radiation critically must be kept as low as reasonably achievable and techniques such as collimation, or aligning the structures of interest, as well as limiting the radiation per image are used to minimize exposure.[18]

The "sniff test" or diaphragmatic fluoroscopy has long been considered the gold-standard for the diagnosis of diaphragm paralysis.[19] Diaphragm paralysis is diagnosed when paradoxic movement is identified on fluoroscopy during sniffing or deep inspiration.[20] Paradoxic motion does correlate favorably with symptomatic improvement on diaphragm plication.[21]

Fluoroscopy has high sensitivity but may have false positives. During normal respiration, the diaphragms contract and descend. Even in healthy patients without dysfunction, the diaphragms are

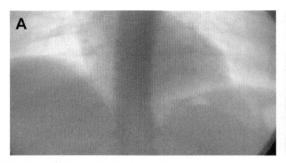
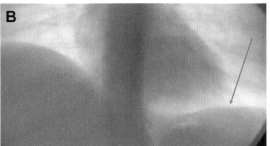

Fig. 3. Sniff test with images captured at end expiration (*A*) and with inspiration (*B*) leading to contraction, flattening, and caudal displacement of the left diaphragm. Diaphragmatic flattening and caudal displacement marked by *red arrow* on the left side of the image. (*Courtesy of* Dr. Tom McLaren.)

asymmetric at rest, the right hemidiaphragm projecting superior to the left because of the underlying liver. In addition, the diaphragms may be slightly offset with their motion thus underscoring the importance of achieving a well-timed and instructed study. The test may be falsely negative in patients with diaphragmatic weakness or incomplete paralysis. In cases of bilateral diaphragm paralysis, it is unusual to find the classic paradoxic movement as the diaphragm may descend due to outward recoil of the diaphragm wall.[8,22]

Computed Tomography Scan

A CT scan is a computerized image that uses narrow beam, serial x-rays that are fired in a circumferential manner. Opposite each x-ray source is a detector and after each complete rotation, the accumulated data is transferred to a computer to create a tomographic image. This single, cross-sectional slice of anatomy can then be stacked

with each subsequent image to form a 3-dimensional image of a patient.[23]

CT scanning is comparatively a newer technology, dating back only to 1971, but has evolved dramatically with improvements in both resolution and speed.[24] Newer lower dose options help to address the concerns of repeated radiation exposure and cancer risk, and the integration of artificial intelligence continues to enhance interpretation and diagnostic accuracy thereby helping to overcome some drawbacks.[25]

CT scans provide highly detailed images and are advantageous in the morphologic assessment of the diaphragms. The diaphragms can be comparatively evaluated for shape, position, and thickness, which is useful in the diagnosis of eventration or paralysis and can provide data as to potential causes. Abnormalities such as tumors or cysts may be delineated and, in some cases, have features that can assist in diagnosis—that is, lipomatous components for liposarcoma.[26] CT

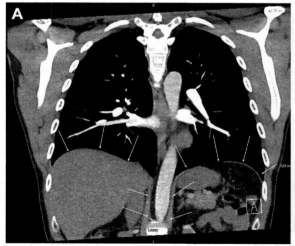
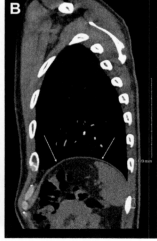

Fig. 4. Coronal (*A*) computed tomography (CT) scan view of the diaphragm demonstrating a normal esophageal hiatus denoted by the arrow. A sagittal (*B*) CT scan of the chest, demonstrating the left hemidiaphragm. (*Courtesy of* Dr. Tom McLaren.)

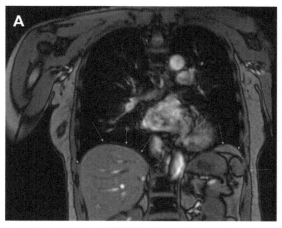
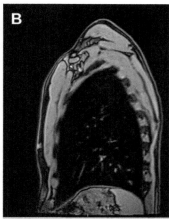

Fig. 5. Coronal (*A*) and sagittal (*B*) MRI of the chest and abdomen; the diaphragm is noted with the arrow. The normal diaphragm is just a thin band with a low intensity on both T1-weighted and T2-weighted images. (*Courtesy of* Dr. Tom McLaren.)

scans have been well established in the trauma literature as providing a useful role in identifying both penetrating diaphragmatic injury and blunt rupture. The pathognomonic signs will be discussed in great detail in Chapter: Management of Traumatic Diaphragmatic Injuries.[27] Finally, CT scan is the imaging of choice for diaphragmatic hernias by providing a view of the location, size, and anatomic contents as well as possible complications.[28,29]

MRI

MRI leverages the magnetic properties of cells to create images. Hydrogen protons throughout the body exist in randomly aligned axes. A magnetic field will create alignment of cells and when a radio frequency is added, cells resonate differentially. When the radio frequency is turned off, a radio wave is emitted, measured, and translated into cross-sectional images.[30]

MRI eliminates the risk of radiation exposure, provides a wide field of view, 3-dimensional presentation, and a comprehensive morphologic assessment of the diaphragm. The downsides to MRI are namely cost and patient factors—some implantable metal devices are incompatible with MRI and claustrophobia. Other risks include auditory issues secondary to the heating of tissues from the radio frequency field that is created.[31]

Normal MRI appearance of a diaphragm is a thin band spanning the chest with low signal intensity on T1-weighted and T2-weighted images (**Figs. 3–5**).[3,15]A unique benefit is the ability to obtain dynamic imaging, which in the case of the diaphragm permits assessment over the course of a respiratory cycle in multiple planes. Post-processing analysis can provide useful additional information

such as kinetics, degree of movement, and directionality.[8,32]

The applications of MRI for the assessment of the diaphragm are broad. This is a safe choice for congenital diaphragmatic hernias providing anatomic details as to the defect but, in addition, in the assessment of fetal lung volume, organ herniation, and helping predict neonatal survival.[1] Likewise, it is effective for acquired hernias, paralysis, eventration, evaluating primary and secondary tumors, and has been particularly useful in characterizing benign cysts, tumors, or benign tumors.[1]

SUMMARY

A plethora of imaging options exist for the diagnosis of diaphragm pathology. Selecting the right approach to provide either anatomic or functional detail is critical to guiding next steps in patient care.

CLINICS CARE POINTS

- Chest x-ray is the most commonly performed modality and can provide a static evaluation of chest morphology.

- A CT scan while also static can provide highly detailed images that is advantageous in evaluating the shape, position, thickness and and pathologies of the diaphragm, in partiucular hernias and tumors.

- Functional studies such as ultrasound, fluoroscopy and MRI can provide both anatomic and functional detail that can aid in the determination of palsy or paralysis.

DISCLOSURE

I am a consultant for Intuitive surgical, BMS, Genentech and Merck. I give talks on behalf of Intuitive, BMS and ASCO. None of these are pertinent to the contents of this chapter.

REFERENCES

1. Cicero G, Mazziotti S, Blandino A, et al. Magnetic resonance imaging of the diaphragm: from normal to pathologic findings. J Clin Imaging Sci 2020; 10(1). https://doi.org/10.25259/JCIS_138_2019.
2. Abbey-Mensah GN, Waite S, Reede D, et al. Diaphragm appearance: A clue to the diagnosis of pulmonary and extrapulmonary pathology. Curr Probl Diag Radiol 2017;46:47–62.
3. Chavhan GB, Babyn PS, Cohen RA, et al. Multimodality imaging of the pediatric diaphragm: Anatomy and pathologic conditions. Radiographics 2010;30: 1797–817.
4. Jones CM, Buchlak QD, Oakden-Rayner L, et al. Chest radiographs and machine learning – Past, present and future. J Med Imaging Radiat Oncol 2021;65(5):538–44.
5. Gefter W, Post BA, Hatabu H. Commonly Missed Findings on Chest Radiographs. Chest 2023;163(3):650–61.
6. Verhey PT, Gosselin MV, Primack SL, et al. Differentiating diaphragmatic paralysis and eventration. Acad Radiol 2007;14(4):420–5.
7. Sandstrom CK, Stern EJ. Diaphragm hernias: a spectrum of radiographic appearances. Curr Prob Diag Radiol 2011;40(3):95–115.
8. Laghi FA, Saad M, Shaikh H. Ultrasound and non-ultrasound imaging techniques in the assessment of diaphragm dysfunction. BMC Pulm Med 2021; 21(85). https://doi.org/10.1186/s12890-021-01441-6.
9. Wait JL, Nahormek PA, Yost WT, et al. Diaphragmatic thickness-lung volume relationship in vivo. J Appl Physiol 1989;67(4):1560–8.
10. Au A, Zwank M. Physics and Technical Facts for the Beginner. Sonography. American College of Emergency Physicians. https://www.acep.org/sonoguide/basic/ultrasound-physics-and-technical-facts-for-the-beginner.
11. Goligher EC, Dres M, Fan Eddy, et al. Mechanical Ventilation-induced Diaphragm Atrophy Strongly Impacts Clinical Outcome. American J Resp and Crit Care 2018;197(2). https://doi.org/10.1164/rccm.201703-0536OC.
12. Boussuges A, Gole Y, Blanc P. Diaphragmatic motion studied by m-mode ultrasonography: methods, reproducibility, and normal values. Chest 2009;135(2): 391–400.
13. Ricoy J, Rodriguez-Nunez N, Alvarez-Dobano JM, et al. Diaphragmatic dysfunction. Pulmonology 2019;25(4):223–35.
14. Boon AJ, Harper CJ, Ghahfarokhi LS, et al. Two-dimensional ultrasound imaging of the diaphragm: quantitative values in normal subjects. Muscle Nerve 2013;47(6):884–9.
15. Kharma N. Dysfunction of the diaphragm: Imaging as a diagnostic tool. Curr Opin Pulm Med 2013;19: 394–8.
16. Levine MS, Rubesin SE, Laufer I. Barium studies in modern radiology: do they have a role? Radiology 2009;250:18–22.
17. Shalom NE, Grong GX, Auster M. Fluoroscopy: An essential diagnostic modality in the age of high-resolution cross-sectional imaging. World J Radiol 2020;12(10):213–30.
18. Bushberg JT, Seibert JA, Leidholdt EM, et al. The essential physics of medical imaging. 3rd edition. Philadelphia, PA: Lippincott Williams & Wilkins; 2012. http://books.google.com/books?id=RKcTgTqeniwC&printsec=frontcover&dq=The+Essential+Physics+of+Medical+Imaging,+3rd+Edition&hl=en&sa=X&ei=L-tlVLbCIs6zyASEioK4Bw&ved=0CDIQ6AEwAA#v=onepage&q=TheEssentialPhysicsofMedicalImaging,3rdEdition&f=false.
19. Lloyd T, Tang Y, Benson M, et al. Diaphragmatic paralysis: the use of M mode ultrasound for diagnosis in adults. Spinal Cord 2006;505–8. https://doi.org/10.1038/sj.sc.3101889.
20. Reed JC. Chapter 6L elevated diaphragm, chest radiology. 7th Edition. Elsevier; 2019. p. 63–70. https://doi.org/10.1016/B978-0-323-49831-9.00006-3.
21. Patel D, Berry M, Bhandari P, et al. Paradoxical motion on sniff test predicts greater improvement following diaphragm plication. An Thorac Surg 2021;111(6):1820–6.
22. Newsom-Davis JG, Loh M, Casson M. Diaphragm function and alveolar hypoventilation. Q J Med 1976;177:87–100.
23. NIH Computed Tomography https://www.nibib.nih.gov/science-education/science-topics/computed-tomography-ct.
24. Schulz RA, Stein JA, Pelc NJ. How CT happened: the early development of medical computed tomography. J Med Imag 2021;8(5):052110.
25. Grenier PA, Brun AL, Mellot F. The Potential Role of Artificial Intelligence in Lung Cancer Screening Using Low-Dose Computed Tomography. Diagnostics 2022; 12(10):2435.
26. Viragh KA, Cherneykin S, Oomen R, et al. Primary liposarcoma of the diaphragm: a rare intra-abdominal mass. Radiol Case Rep 2017;12(1): 136–40.
27. Panda A, Kumar A, Gamanagatti S, et al. Traumatic diaphragmatic injury: a review of CT signs and the difference between blunt and penetrating injury. Diag Interv Radiol 2014;20(2):121–8.
28. Sodhi KS, Virmani V, Sandhu MS, et al. Multi detector CT Imaging of Abdominal and Diaphragmatic

Hernias: Pictorial Essay. Indian J Surg 2015;77(2): 104–10.

29. Eren S, Ciris F. Diaphragmatic hernia: diagnostic approaches with review of the literature. Eur J Radiol 2005;54(3):448–59.

30. Berger A. Magnetic Resonance Imaging. BMC (Biomed Chromatogr) 2002;324(7328):35.

31. Ghadimi M, Sapra A. Magnetic resonance imaging contraindications. StatPears; 2023. https://www.ncbi.nlm.nih.gov/books/NBK551669/.

32. Gierada DS, Curtin JJ, Erickson SJ, et al. Diaphragmatic motion: Fast gradient-recalled-echo MR imaging in healthy subjects. Radiology 1995; 194:879–84.

Reconstructive Techniques for Diaphragm Resection

Dina Al Rameni, MD[a], Stephanie G. Worrell, MD[a,b],*

KEYWORDS

- Diaphragm • Diaphragmatic reconstruction • Synthetic mesh • Primary repair

KEY POINTS

- Various diaphragmatic and nondiaphragmatic abnormalities may necessitate surgery to reconstruct the diaphragm.
- The surgical approach for diaphragmatic reconstruction involves thoracic, abdominal, or combined thoracoabdominal approaches.
- The utilization of minimally invasive techniques, such as video-assisted thoracoscopic, laparoscopic, and robotic approached are becoming increasingly common.
- Optimal management of diaphragmatic defects involves primary repair when the reconstruction achieves a tension-free state. In other circumstances, the consideration of prosthetic replacement or autologous flaps becomes imperative.
- When repairing or reconstructing the diaphragm, it is crucial to preserve the major branches of the phrenic nerves to maintain functional integrity.

INTRODUCTION

The diaphragm can be involved by thoracic or abdominal tumors by direct extension. In some instances, en-bloc resection of the diaphragm and reconstruction with prosthetic material is necessary. Preserving the physiologic function of the diaphragm and ensuring adequate respiratory status are essential after diaphragm resection. Surgical 764550aL access to the diaphragm can be achieved through 3 approaches: trans-thoracic, transabdominal, or a combination of both. Defects can be approximated primarily, reconstructed with bioprosthetic or synthetic mesh, or bridged with autologous muscle flap. This article explores the various surgical techniques for diaphragm reconstruction.

PRE-PROCEDURAL PLANNING

When choosing a surgical approach for the diaphragm, several factors must be taken into consideration. These factors include the specific portion of the diaphragm requiring exposure, the presence of surrounding organs and structures that could impede this exposure (such as associated thoracic or abdominal abnormalities), the intended repair, and the surgeon's personal preference and level of experience. Comprehensive preoperative planning and the careful selection of a surgical approach aid in minimizing the length and quantity of incisions, as well as reducing the potential for resulting restrictive respiratory dysfunction.

ANATOMY

The diaphragm is considered to be the second most important muscle after the heart. The diaphragm is anatomically made up of muscle that originates from the chest wall and coalesces in the central tendon (Chapter 1). The blood supply is primarily from the phrenic artery and vein centrally and the intercostal vessels along the periphery, **Fig. 1.**

[a] Divison of Cardiothoracic Surgery, Department of Surgery, University of Arizona- College of Medicine, 1501 North Campbell Avenue, Room #4302, PO Box 245071, Tucson, AZ 85724, USA; [b] University of Arizona, 1501 North Campbell Avenue, Tucson, AZ 85724, USA
* Corresponding author. University of Arizona, 1501 North Campbell Avenue, Tucson, AZ 85724.
E-mail address: sworrell@arizona.edu
Twitter: @DinaSRamini (D.A.R.); @Sgworrell (S.G.W.)

Thorac Surg Clin 34 (2024) 127–131
https://doi.org/10.1016/j.thorsurg.2024.01.001
1547-4127/24/© 2024 Elsevier Inc. All rights reserved.

thoracic.theclinics.com

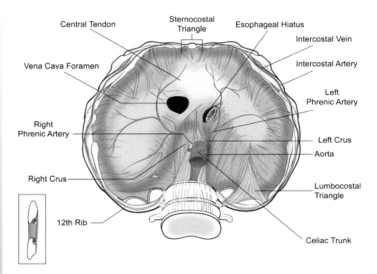

Central Tendon

Sternocostal Triangle

Esophageal Hiatus

Intercostal Vein

Intercostal Artery

Vena Cava Foramen

Left Phrenic Artery

Right Phrenic Artery

Left Crus

Aorta

Right Crus

Lumbocostal Triangle

12th Rib

Celiac Trunk

Fig. 1. The blood supply is primarily from the phrenic artery and vein centrally and the intercostal vessels along the periphery. (Reference: David J. Finley MD, Nadeem R. Abu-Rustum MD, Dennis S. Chi MD and Raja Flores MD Thoracic Surgery Clinics, 2009-11-01, Volume 19, Issue 4, Pages 531-535, Copyright © 2009 Elsevier Inc.)

SURGICAL APPROACH

Trans-abdominal Approach

The abdominal approach, via laparotomy or laparoscopy, is preferred in patients with thoracoabdominal trauma and diaphragmatic rupture undergoing simultaneous diagnostic laparoscopy/laparotomy for abdominal pathology. Additionally, this approach is ideal for management of anterolateral diaphragmatic hernias and congenital diaphragmatic hernias in children.[1]

The exposure and operative positioning should be selected based on the location of the tumor or defect requiring repair. The left diaphragm is easily exposed with this approach, but the right diaphragm is difficult to access through the abdomen and even more difficult to reconstruct. Additionally, while laparotomy is an effective surgical technique, it is important to consider potential drawbacks. These may include longer recovery time, increased postoperative pain, and the potential for complications such as infection, bleeding, or damage to nearby organs.[2,3] Robotic and laparoscopic approaches may be feasible with smaller tumors or defects and have potential benefits such as reduced postoperative pain, shorter hospital stays, and faster recovery compared to traditional open surgery.[2,3]

Thoracic Approach

Large intrathoracic tumors or tumors that involve other intrathoracic organs are best approached through the chest. Additionally, when extensive abdominal adhesions make safe abdominal access challenging, the preferred method to access the diaphragm is through the chest, either via thoracotomy or thoracoscopy. This approach is commonly used for treating conditions such as diaphragmatic eventration and chronic diaphragmatic hernias. Typically, patients are positioned in a decubitus position on the side opposite to the side of repair.[4] There is a growing interest in robot-assisted thoracoscopic diaphragmatic reconstruction. The robot is particularly advantageous as it allows for enhanced optics and operative ergonomics, coupled with better instruments articulation.[5] For robot-assisted thoracoscopic approach, CO_2 insufflation provides expansion of the thoracic cavity by a contralateral shift of the mediastinum, expansion of the intercostal spaces, and, most importantly, caudal displacement of the diaphragm. Resultant enlarged intrathoracic space facilitates the visualization and exposure of the anatomy and overall conduct of the operation[6] (Fig. 2).

Thoracoabdominal Approach

The thoracoabdominal approach offers the advantage of providing access to both the chest and

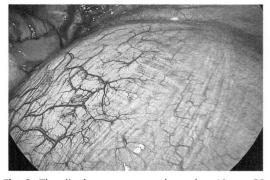

Fig. 2. The diaphragm as seen through a 10-mm 30-degree thoracoscopic camera.

abdomen, resulting in improved exposure for challenging cases involving the spine and thoracoabdominal aorta. The left thoracoabdominal approach is particularly beneficial for complex esophagogastric procedures, while the right approach is useful for traumatic liver and diaphragmatic injuries.

Typically, the incision starts from the umbilicus and extends toward the costal arch, continuing along the seventh or eighth intercostal space in the chest wall. Alternatively, it can begin with a thoracotomy and proceed with a laparotomy as needed. Transection of the abdominal muscles, chondrocostal cartilage, and thoracic muscles (serratus anterior and latissimus dorsi) allows for improved access. The incision can be extended dorsally as required.

RECONSTRUCTION TECHNIQUES
Primary Repair

Primary repair of diaphragmatic defects is feasible when there is sufficient tissue available that can be brought together without tension, ensuring an airtight seal of the chest cavity without causing paradoxic chest movement.[7] The muscular nature of the diaphragm allows it to tolerate wide incisions without compromising its function. The edges of the diaphragm are typically approximated using interrupted, running, or horizontal mattress sutures.[8] Depending on the thickness of the muscle at the area of closure, the suture can be buttressed with felt pledgets to improve the strength of the closure. The key principle is to take full-thickness bites while avoiding injury to structures beneath the diaphragm. In cases of running sutures, a second running suture layer is an option to provide an additional seal.[9] Meticulous attention must be devoted to the inferior vena cava (IVC), descending thoracic aorta, and the supra-hepatic veins during reconstruction.

Repair Using Bioprosthetic or Synthetic Mesh

Diaphragm reconstruction using bioprosthetic or synthetic mesh offers the necessary strength and impermeability.

Examples of synthetic meshes used in diaphragmatic repair.

- Polytetrafluoroethylene (PTFE Gore-Tex, Gore&Assoc, Arizona, USA): 2 mm thickness, easy to handle.
- GORE DUALMESH has a dual-surface material that promotes tissue in-growth while minimizing attachment to abdominal viscera.

- Mersilene polyester fiber mesh (Ethicon, Somerville, NJ, USA): non-absorbable and permeable prosthetic
- Prolene double-filamented polypropylene mesh (Ethicon, Somerville, NJ, USA)
- Marlex polypropylene monofilamented fiber mesh (Davol, Cranston, RI)
- Polyethylene methylmethacrylate sandwich flaps have also shown excellent functional and cosmetic outcomes.

Biologic mesh should be used with caution as the absorption can leave a future diaphragmatic defect. However, in areas of contamination, it offers an alternative if primary repair is not achievable. Biologic mesh utilizes a technology where cells and immunogenic properties are removed, allowing the host epithelium to easily re-colonize the scaffold of the basal membrane. Consequently, the biologic mesh in theory maintains the strength and integrity of the repair while undergoing remodeling.

Examples of biological meshes used in diaphragmatic repair[10,11]

- Bovine pericardium
- Acellular porcine dermal collagen (Permacol Covidien, AG, USA)
- Acellular human dermis (AlloDerm, Lifecell Corporation, Branchburg, NJ, USA)

Once the diaphragm resection is completed, the mesh is typically sewn to the rim of the diaphragm using continuous runs of large non-absorbable sutures. The edges of the mesh are then secured with interrupted runs of monofilament non-absorbable sutures to the involved ribs, if necessary. It is a common practice to over-correct the reconstruction by placing the prosthesis in a lower position than the native diaphragm, giving it a steeper shape. Therefore, the goal should be to position the anchoring stitches slightly higher than one would expect to get a slightly more physiologic elevated position. If the diaphragm is sutured below the ninth rib where there is no attachment to the sternum, this might result in an unstable diaphragm and subsequently respiratory compromise.[12]

The most common site of diaphragmatic patch dehiscence is the left posterior costophrenic corner.[13] This often occurs in cases where extensive diaphragmatic resections leave no viable tissue for securing the stitches and patch. It is recommend leaving, if oncolocigcally feasible, a small rim (maximum 2 cm) of autologous diaphragm along the edge to preserve a secure anchoring space for the mesh. Placing stay stitches on the diaphragmatic rim after resection is crucial to prevent muscular retraction.

Reconstruction with Autologous Muscle Flap

Autologous reconstruction using muscle pedicled flaps, including the transverse rectus abdominis muscle technique, external oblique muscle flap, and latissimus dorsi muscle (LDM) reverse flap, provides the advantage of utilizing vascularized tissue without the need for a permanent foreign body, reducing the risk of potential infections. However, the harvesting technique is typically complex and time-consuming, increasing the likelihood of morbidity and complications at the donor site. Among these options, the technique described by Bedini and colleagues has shown consistent success when applied in mesothelioma resection or for large sarcomas.[7] The LDM of the non-dominant arm has been described to repair diaphragmatic defects, but as a "reverse" flap, relying on secondary blood supply from the perforating lumbar vessels rather than primary inflow from the dominant thoracodorsal artery.[14] It is harvested using an axillary Z-incision, taking care to preserve the muscle tension by placing sutures at defined muscle length. Retraction or shortening of the LDM during insertion would compromise the contractile strength of the transplanted muscle. The LDM is fully elevated, except for the neurovascular bundle, which remains intact until the recipient vessels and nerve are prepared for microanastomosis. After preparing the diaphragm defect, the LDM is transferred to the desired location. If used as a free flap, microsurgical vascular anastomosis is performed with the internal mammary artery. Alternatively, the LDM can be utilized as a rotational flap if it can reach the target site without tension.[15]

OUTCOMES & COMPLICATIONS

Studies have shown that there were no notable disparities identified in terms of complication rates or reconstruction methods when considering the various meshes employed for diaphragmatic and chest wall reconstructions[7] Therefore, mesh selection is at the discretion of the surgeon and often based on experience and personal preference.

Iatrogenic diaphragmatic hernias are among the most prevalent postoperative complications and are often attributed to technical errors during the reconstruction process. Regarding mesh complications, it has been reported that some mesh have the ability to migrate into the abdominal cavity and erode or perforate intrabdominal organs.[16] Overall, this is a rare complication, but a high degree of suspicion and re-assessment of the mesh position over time is important.

Vascular injury at the time of resection and reconstruction can occur, appropriate knowledge of the anatomy and care of the phrenic vessels as well as IVC, hepatic veins, and aorta are important.

CLINICS CARE POINTS

- Optimal management of diaphragmatic defects involves primary repair when the reconstruction achieves a tension-free approximation of the defect's edges. In all other circumstances, the consideration of prosthetic replacement or autologous flaps is imperative, regardless of the size of the defect.
- Diaphragmatic reconstruction can be approached via the abdomen, the chest, or through a combined approach.
- Iatrogenic hernias are among the most prevalent postoperative complications and are often attributed to technical errors during the reconstruction process.

DISCLOSURE

The authors have nothing to disclose.

REFERENCES

1. Henderson RD, Marryatt GV. Reflux control following gastric surgery. Can J Surg 1984;27(1):17–9.
2. Kaltoft B, Gögenur I, Rosenberg J. Reduced length of stay and convalescence in laparoscopic vs open sigmoid resection with traditional care: a double blinded randomized clinical trial. Colorectal Dis 2011;13(6):e123–30.
3. Butler EK, Mills BM, Arbabi S, et al. Laparoscopy Compared With Laparotomy for the Management of Pediatric Blunt Abdominal Trauma. J Surg Res 2020;251:303–10.
4. Graham DR, Kaplan D, Evans CC, et al. Diaphragmatic plication for unilateral diaphragmatic paralysis: a 10-year experience. Ann Thorac Surg 1990; 49(2):248–51 [discussion 252].
5. Zwischenberger BA, Kister N, Zwischenberger JB, et al. Laparoscopic Robot-Assisted Diaphragm Plication. Ann Thorac Surg 2016;101(1):369–71.
6. Gritsiuta AI, Gordon M, Bakhos CT, et al. Minimally Invasive Diaphragm Plication for Acquired Unilateral Diaphragm Paralysis: A Systematic Review. Innovations 2022;17(3):180–90.
7. Kuwahara H, Salo J, Tukiainen E. Diaphragm reconstruction combined with thoraco-abdominal wall

reconstruction after tumor resection. J Plast Surg Hand Surg 2018;52(3):172–7.

8. Matsuda Y, Hoshikawa Y. [Traumatic Diaphragmatic Injury]. Kyobu Geka 2022;75(10):872–7.

9. Demos DS, Berry MF, Backhus LM, et al. Video-assisted thoracoscopic diaphragm plication using a running suture technique is durable and effective. J Thorac Cardiovasc Surg 2017;153(5):1182–8.

10. Antoniou SA, Pointner R, Granderath FA, et al. The Use of Biological Meshes in Diaphragmatic Defects - An Evidence-Based Review of the Literature. Front Surg 2015;2:56.

11. Finley DJ, Abu-Rustum NR, Chi DS, et al. Reconstructive techniques after diaphragm resection. Thorac Surg Clin 2009;19(4):531–5.

12. Abdel Jalil R, Abou Chaar MK, Al-Qudah O, et al. Chest wall and diaphragm reconstruction; a technique not well established in literature - case report. J Cardiothorac Surg 2021;16(1):196.

13. Solli P, Brandolini J, Pardolesi A, et al. Diaphragmatic and pericardial reconstruction after surgery for malignant pleural mesothelioma. J Thorac Dis 2018;10(Suppl 2):S298–303.

14. McConkey MO, Temple CLF, McFadden S, et al. Autologous diaphragm reconstruction with the pedicled latissimus dorsi flap. J Surg Oncol 2006;94(3):248–51.

15. Ninkovic M, Öfner D. Reconstruction of Large Full-Thickness Abdominal Wall Defects Using a Free Functional Latissimus Dorsi Muscle. Front Surg 2022;9:853639.

16. Lee S, Hong SY, Son JA, et al. A Complication of Diaphragm Repair Using a Gore-Tex (Expanded Polytetrafluorethylene) Membrane: A Case Report. J Chest Surg 2022;55(2):171–3.

Diaphragmatic Defects in Infants
Acute Management and Repair

Robert J. Vandewalle, MD, MBA[a],*, Lawrence E. Greiten, MD, MSc[b]

KEYWORDS

- Congenital diaphragmatic hernia (CDH) • Surgical management
- Extracorporeal membrane oxygenation • Pulmonary hypertension

KEY POINTS

- Congenital diaphragmatic hernia (CDH) is complex and should be treated by multidisciplinary teams designed for their care.
- Treatment is focused on pulmonary hypoplasia, pulmonary hypertension, and cardiac dysfunction.
- When medical management fails, extracorporeal membrane oxygenation (ECMO) can be considered. Repair of the CDH early during the ECMO course seems to improve mortality.
- The choice of surgical repair should consider the patient's physiologic status, the surgeon's familiarity, and the pros/cons of each technique.

INTRODUCTION

Congenital diaphragmatic hernias (CDHs) technically encompass posterolateral defects (Bochdalek), anteromedial defects (Morgagni), and central defects (such as those associated with pentalogy of Cantrell) that are present at birth. Bochdalek hernias account for greater than 95% of CDHs.[1–3] Therefore, the focus of this article will be on Bochdalek hernias. For brevity, the term CDH will be used in reference to Bochdalek hernias. The incidence of CDH is reported to be approximately 1 in 3500 in live births, but this does not account for pregnancies that undergo either elective or spontaneous abortion.[1,3–5]

CDH encompasses a wide variety of presentations from minimally symptomatic to fatal. It is this variability in presentation that has made optimization of care difficult and the nidus for developing multidisciplinary care and multicenter collaboration toward the goal of improving outcomes in neonates with CDH. Two international organizations, the CDH Study Group (CDHSG) and the Extracorporeal Life Support Organization (ELSO), provide resources for patient care, ongoing research, and multicenter collaboration. Participation in these organizations is imperative for institutions that care for the CDH population. Despite multiple advancements in care, the mortality rate of liveborn neonates with CDH has remained approximately 20% to 30% since the 1990s.[6,7]

The embryologic derangements in CDH are not completely understood. In general, the development of the diaphragm is believed to involve four structures: the septum transversum (central), the pleuroperitoneal folds (posterolateral), dorsal mesentery (around esophagus), and thoracic body wall.[8] Other embryologic defects of the chest have also been proposed.[8] Ultimately, CDH results in a posterior defect with herniation of variable amounts of abdominal viscera into the ipsilateral thoracic cavity and regional hypoplasia involving the ipsilateral lung and to a lesser extent the heart/contralateral lung.[6,9–11] Alterations in the pulmonary vascular bed including

[a] Department of Surgery, University of Arkansas for Medical Sciences/Arkansas Children's Hospital, 1 Children's Way, Slot 844, Little Rock, AR 72202, USA; [b] Department of Surgery, University of Arkansas for Medical Sciences/Arkansas Children's Hospital, 1 Children's Way, Slot 677, Little Rock, AR 72202, USA
* Corresponding author.
E-mail address: RVandewalle@uams.edu

Thorac Surg Clin 34 (2024) 133–145
https://doi.org/10.1016/j.thorsurg.2024.01.003
1547-4127/24/© 2024 Elsevier Inc. All rights reserved.

hypoplasia/decreased vascular branching and increased muscle within the media of the pulmonary arteries lead to pulmonary hypertension.[6,12,13] Approximately 85% of CDH occurs on the left side. Interestingly, only about 20% of patients have a hernia sac, regardless of the side of presentation and this has been found to confer a milder disease process in systematic reviews.[1,2,14,15]

CDH is termed "isolated" when it is not associated with a known genetic mutation or other congenital defects. Approximately 60% of CDH are isolated. Concomitant congenital heart disease is the most common form of "non-isolated" CDH and occurs in 50% of cases.[2,3,16] When associated congenital heart disease is present, there is an increase in mortality depending on the severity of the cardiac lesion.[6,16,17] The most common associated aneuploidy is trisomy 18.[3,8] Additional proposed genetic causes are numerous, but approximately 80% of cases have no established genetic etiology.[3]

Approximately two-third of all CDH are diagnosed by the second trimester of pregnancy, typically by screening ultrasound.[6,14,18–20] Prenatal detection allows for a multidisciplinary approach to management of patients with CDH and their families. This team should include maternal–fetal medicine, neonatology, radiology, and the potential operating surgeon. Counseling should include prenatal guidance regarding morbidity, mortality, timing/location of delivery, and other treatment choices available to the family. After the diagnosis of CDH has been made prenatally, patients should be counseled on the need for genetic testing and a comprehensive fetal ultrasound/fetal echocardiogram.[6] These diagnostic studies aid in risk stratification of the fetus.

The observed-to-expected lung-to-head ratio (O/E LHR) is the most commonly used measurement when assessing CDH severity.[21,22] In left-sided CDH, the O/E LHR as well as the presence/absence of the liver within thoracic cavity (ie, "liver up") has been shown to predict survival.[22,23] Grading of CDH severity and survival is classically described as follows:[6,14,22]

- Mild: O/E LHR 36% to 45% with liver down or greater than 45% regardless of liver position (>75% survival)
- Moderate: O/E LHR 26% to 35% with liver down or 36% to 45% with liver up (survival 40%–60%)
- Severe: O/E LHR 15% to 25% (survival 20%–30%)
- Extremely Severe: O/E LHR less than 15% (survival <5%)

There are multiple techniques used to calculate the O/E LHR which can limit reproducibility.[20,24] Fetal MRI has been adopted by many institutions, but the indices used and techniques used to calculate them have yet to be standardized.[20,24,25] Right-sided CDH more commonly have liver herniation, which may not be as accurate of a predictor for morbidity/mortality as compared with left.[26,27]

Finally, fetal endoscopic tracheal occlusion is a surgical option provided by select fetal centers of excellence in the United States and Europe. This technique involves placement of an occlusive balloon in the fetus' airway to promote growth of the hypoplastic lung.[28] At this time, patients with an O/E LHR less than 25% are considered candidates for the procedure, which takes place between 27 and 30 weeks gestation.[23,29] There are multiple contraindications to performing this procedure, but any patient seen with the appropriate indications should be considered for referral.

ACUTE MANAGEMENT

Children with a prenatal diagnosis of CDH should be delivered at an institution with the capacity to manage their immediate needs.[30] The acute care is focused on the management of three major factors: pulmonary hypoplasia, pulmonary hypertension, and cardiac dysfunction. Single institution and national/international care guidelines are available for reference.[6,31–37] At this time, there is no proven benefit to early term versus full term delivery.[38]

Initial Resuscitation

Respiratory support immediately after birth focuses on maintaining adequate oxygenation and ventilation without inducing iatrogenic trauma to the hypoplastic lung. In stable low-risk patients at the appropriate institution, this can be accomplished with supplemental oxygen via a nasal cannula.[39] Outside of these scenarios, intubation immediately after birth should be completed. The avoidance of noninvasive positive pressure modalities such as continuous positive airway pressure and manual bagging is imperative. Swallowed air can further distend viscera within the chest, worsening pulmonary function. Pneumothorax is a known negative predictor for survival in CDH.[5,40] Similarly, gastric decompression should be completed early in the resuscitative phase.[5]

Intravenous and intra-arterial access (typically via the umbilical vessels) is obtained, and both pre- and post-ductal oxygen saturation monitors are placed. In the setting of hypotension, judicious use of isotonic fluid boluses before initiating vasopressor therapy is required to prevent volume overload and/or exacerbate cardiac dysfunction. Abdominal/chest x-ray(s) confirm the diagnosis as well as acceptable placement of invasive lines/tubes. Echocardiogram within the first 12 to 24 hours of life determines the degree of pulmonary hypertension as well as ventricular function, and repeat examinations are completed as needed.[13,41,42] Adequate sedation and minimizing stimulation can also prevent exacerbation of pulmonary hypertension.

Ventilatory Support

Ventilatory strategies in CDH are based on lung-protective concepts (ie, "gentle ventilation") as well as permissive hypercapnia. Initial preductal oxygen saturations $\geq 85\%$ are typically considered acceptable if clinical signs of adequate perfusion are maintained.[33,36,43] Historically, patients were immediately placed on an Fio_2 of 1.0 after intubation. However, this ventilator strategy has been questioned relating to the long-term side effects of high oxygen supplementation. In fact, this strategy may be associated with lower survival and higher extracorporeal membrane oxygenation (ECMO) utilization.[44,45] It is reasonable to either wean Fio_2 lower than 1.0 after initial intubation or start at a lower Fio_2 and titrate as needed clinically.[36,43,45] Hypercapnia is considered tolerable for $Paco_2 \leq 65$ to 70 mm Hg as long as arterial pH ≥ 7.25 is maintained with good clinical markers for perfusion.[33,46] Volume- or pressure-controlled conventional ventilation strategies are acceptable. Most CDH-specific protocols limit peak inspiratory pressures to ≤ 25 to 28 cm H_2O and tidal volumes are initially targeted at ~ 4 mL/kg to compensate for the hypoplastic lung.[33,36,37,46] The VICI-trial compared conventional ventilation with high-frequency oscillatory ventilation (HFOV) for initial respiratory management in CDH and found similar rates of mortality and bronchopulmonary dysplasia.[47] Although there was no improvement in mortality among ventilation strategies, there was a higher utilization of vasopressors, duration of mechanical ventilation, and ECMO use in the HFOV cohort.[47]

Pulmonary Hypertension

Uncontrolled pulmonary hypertension ultimately results in right heart failure and death. In the CDH population, pulmonary hypertension (CDH-PH) is considered to have both "reversible" and "irreversible" components.[13,48] The reversible components of CDH-PH refer to hyperreactivity of the pulmonary vascular bed and are the targets of medical intervention.[13,48] The irreversible components are those related to paucity of branching of the vascular bed

combined with the hyperplasia of the muscular media layer.[13,48] Pulmonary hypertension reported via echocardiogram is normally categorized as either none, less than two-third systemic pressure (moderate), greater than two-third systemic pressure (severe), or supra-systemic (extreme) based on tricuspid regurgitation jet estimation.[13] Additional factors suggesting CDH-PH on echocardiography include dynamic position of the intraventricular septum and direction of flow through the patent ductus arteriosus (PDA), with right-to-left flow or biphasic flow suggesting significant pulmonary hypertension.[13]

Several agents are available for treatment of CDH-PH. The most common is inhaled nitrous oxide (iNO). Data support the use of iNO in non-CDH neonates with persistent pulmonary hypertension. However, reports in the CDH population are mixed, with some data suggesting it may worsen mortality in the pre-repaired population.[49–51] Similarly, there has been no proven reduction in ECMO utilization for patients with CDH-PH, and current indications for starting iNO are not uniform across institutions.[49–51] A recent paper by Noh and colleagues reported the early use of iNO did not improve mortality or reduce ECMO utilization, further questioning its utility in this patient population.[52] iNO may worsen heart failure in patients with impaired left ventricular function. Sildenafil use has similarly increased in popularity over the last decade, but data on its use are largely limited to single-institution reviews.[53] A clinical trial comparing sildenafil to iNO for treatment of CDH-PH is underway.[54]

Prostaglandin E1 (PGE1) is used in some centers to maintain PDA to manage severe pulmonary hypertension, offload a failing right ventricle, and/or enhance systemic blood through right to left shunting via the PDA.[42,55] PGE1 is used extensively in the setting of congenital cardiac defects, but its use in CDH is limited to small retrospective studies.[13,55] Bosentan, epoprostenol, and treprostinil are also agents that have been described for the treatment of CDH-PH, although data are limited.[13]

Ventricular Dysfunction

Concomitant ipsilateral and possible contralateral ventricular hypoplasia with resultant ventricular dysfunction can occur in CDH.[41,42,56] Ventricular, typically diastolic, dysfunction is a known marker for disease severity.[41,42] In the setting of systemic hypotension, judicious use of isotonic fluid boluses is imperative to simultaneously improve perfusion while preventing worsening pulmonary/cardiac function. In the absence of clinical signs of hypovolemia or if hypotension is persistent after fluid administration, additional medical adjuncts should be instituted. The choice of agent(s) should be guided by echocardiographic results and clinical parameters with focus on pulmonary hypertension and systemic cardiovascular status. Typically, dobutamine or epinephrine is first-line agents in patients with reduced ventricular function.[6,42] For those patients with systemic hypotension and retained ventricular function, norepinephrine or vasopressin can be considered.[6,42] There is some evidence that vasopressin is effective at improving both systemic hypotension and CDH-PH but can cause hyponatremia.[57,58]

Milrinone is an inotrope with lusitropic effects. This agent has been used both for treatment of CDH-PH when iNO is ineffective and ventricular dysfunction. A pilot study for its use in CDH is underway.[41,42,56] Milrinone can induce hypotension and has a prolonged half-life of 2 hours.

Finally, when all medical interventions fail, ECMO can be considered but remains controversial in the CDH population.[59] Despite significant advances in neonatal care over the last several decades, the survival of patients with CDH requiring ECMO remains only about 50%.[60] In addition, the indications, contraindications, and choice of ECMO modality (ie, venoarterial vs venovenous) are variable among institutions.[61,62] Considerations for ECMO therapy in the setting of CDH include but are not limited to, persistently low preductal SpO_2, persistently elevated oxygen index, refractory hypoxemia/acidosis, and unacceptably high ventilatory requirements.[61,62]

Before the initiation of ECMO therapy, additional patient-specific factors must be considered within the context of a multidisciplinary team aligned with the families' goals of care. Children with complex/unrepairable cardiac defects and lethal chromosomal anomalies are generally not considered candidates for ECMO.[61] Children with CDH and congenital heart disease causing single-ventricle physiology have are reported survival to discharge of 16%.[16] The presence of a grade III/IV intraventricular hemorrhage is also considered by most to be a contraindication to ECMO therapy.[61,63]

There is no tool/metric available to accurately predict which patients will not survive despite ECMO therapy. The lowest $Paco_2$ obtained after initial resuscitation is a commonly used metric for ECMO utilization/disease severity in high-risk patients.[20,64] Kim and colleagues reported the use of the SPHERE protocol to try to identify non-survivors within the CDH registry based on early resuscitation metrics.[64] High-risk patients were those with a lowest $Paco_2 \geq 100$ mgHg 2 hours after delivery/resuscitation. Although the high-risk group was associated with more resource utilization, it did not predict survival.[64] The duration of ECMO therapy, including the discussion of withdrawing of care, should be based on individual patient progress.[6,59] ECMO therapy lasting more than 4 weeks with successful decannulation, CDH repair, and survival have been described.[65]

CONTROVERSIES
Timing of Repair

Neonates that improve within days of birth and will not need ECMO (ie, low-risk patients) typically are repaired in the first week of life.[66] Patient stability outweighs timing of surgery in this population.[67] Stability is typically defined as resolution of hypoxia with normalization of blood pressure, clinical evidence of adequate perfusion/oxygen delivery, and stabilization of CDH-PH.[36,66,68,69]

The CDH patient requiring ECMO however is far more complex. After initiation of ECMO, there are three potential options for repair: repair shortly after ECMO initiation (early repair within 48–72 hours), repair later in the ECMO course (late repair), or attempt to complete ECMO therapy prior repair (delayed repair). Repair on ECMO has inherent risks related to bleeding/anticoagulation. The adoption of bivalirudin for ECMO anticoagulation in CDH at some centers seems to improve these risks but needs to be validated.[70] Bivalirudin, a direct thrombin inhibitor historically used for patients with heparin-induced thrombocytopenia, has been used for anticoagulation in both adult and pediatric patients on ECMO.[71–75]

Delayed repair has been shown in multiple single-institution reviews and CDHSG studies to have a potential survival advantage.[62,76,77] However, not all children will successfully wean from ECMO before surgery, leading to either non-repair (fatal) or late repair. Dao and colleagues recently reported their CDHSG registry evaluation of early, late, and delayed repair. Early repair was associated with shorter ECMO therapy, shorter length of stay, and 50% reduction in death rate when compared with late repair.[78] When comparing early versus delayed treatment paradigms (and including patients who do not survive to delayed repair), early repair also had a 50% reduction in mortality rate, but with longer ECMO duration and higher oxygen requirements at discharge.[78] This relationship in mortality reverses when non-repairs are excluded.[78] The investigators postulate that early repair likely salvages patients that would otherwise succumb to their disease.[78] Unfortunately, there is no way to identify which patients will be able to liberate from ECMO before surgery.[78] Our institution reported experiences with early repair in 2010, which compared favorably to CDHSG/ELSO registry data at the time.[79] This continues to be our practice.

SURGICAL TECHNIQUES

Multiple techniques for initial repair of CDH are available to the surgeon. The choice of approach is based on the patient's clinical condition as well as the surgeon's comfort with these techniques. Laparoscopic repair has proven to be difficult due to poor visualization of the hernia defect. Therefore, most CDH are either repaired via laparotomy or thoracoscopically.

Laparotomy

Before starting the procedure, the surgeon must decide if they will be performing a mesh closure versus a myofascial closure if required, as this will alter the incision location (**Fig. 1**). After appropriate anesthesia, the affected side of the abdomen and chest are then elevated with a bump/roll to facilitate the exposure of the lateral aspect of the hernia. The abdomen and chest are prepped and draped.

Common steps

- After completing the laparotomy, the abdominal contents are then gently reduced into the abdomen. The spleen is typically reduced last. Moist gauze and malleable retractors work well to keep the abdominal viscera out of the operative field once reduced. If a hernia sac is encountered, it should be removed in full. The size of the defect is noted and should be recorded according to the CDHSG grading criteria (**Fig. 2**) as well as the size of the ipsilateral lung.[80] Standardized reporting aids in communication, prognostication, and is reportable in the CDHSG registry.[80] Defect size has been correlated with survival.[80]

- Frequently retroperitoneal attachments will be adherent to the posterior leaflet of the hernia defect. These are then mobilized, allowing the diaphragm leaflet to be "unrolled."

- The ability to re-approximate the hernia defect primarily is then assessed. If amenable to a primary repair, tension-free approximation is the goal and can be completed with interrupted permanent sutures in a figure of eight or a horizontal mattress fashion, using generous bites of the diaphragm leaflets (with or without pledgets).

- Commonly, the lateral border of the defect does not have diaphragm overlying the associated rib. In this scenario, the lateral borders of the superior and/or inferior leaflets of the diaphragm are opposed to the adjacent rib with pericostal sutures (ie, passing the suture around the rib after obtaining a bite of the diaphragm leaflet). Any defect not amenable for primary repair requires either mesh closure or a myofascial flap.

- It is common to primarily repair a portion of the diaphragmatic defect (most often medially) in areas where there is no tension to minimize the amount of prosthetic mesh/myofascial flap required for closure.

- Before closing the defect using any technique, a thoracostomy tube can be placed under direct visualization into the thoracic space. The thoracostomy tube is left to water seal to allow for drainage of any resultant fluid collections. There is no evidence that thoracostomy tubes increase the risk of surgical site infection, even with mesh. Thoracostomy tubes are placed at the discretion of the surgeon and the intensivist team caring for the patient, with the understanding that the ipsilateral hypoplastic lung often will not fill the resultant dead space. Placing thoracostomy tubes to suction can injure the lung and create significant mediastinal shift.

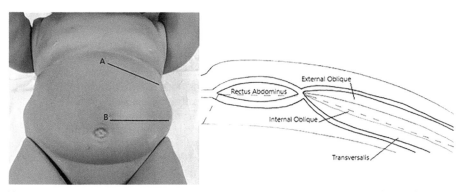

Fig. 1. (*Left*) Laparotomy sites for a left-sided CDH repair if a mesh repair (A) or myofascial flap (B) are chosen. (*Right*) Dissection plane for creation of a myofascial flap for CDH repair.

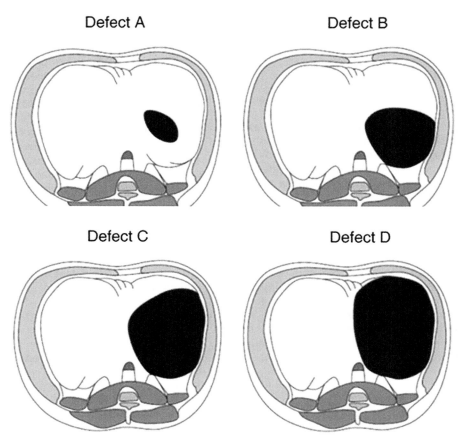

Fig. 2. CDH defect size based on CDHSG standardized reporting. Type A defects are small and surrounded by muscle. Type B defects lack muscle on the chest wall, and the hernia is less than 50% of the hemidiaphragm. Type C defects lack muscle on the chest wall but involve greater than 50% of the diaphragm. Type D defects are complete/near-complete agenesis of the hemidiaphragm. (*From* Lally KP, Lasky RE, Lally PA, Bagolan P, Davis CF, Frenckner BP, Hirschl RM, Langham MR, Buchmiller TL, Usui N, Tibboel D, Wilson JM; Congenital Diaphragmatic Hernia Study Group. Standardized reporting for congenital diaphragmatic hernia–an international consensus. J Pediatr Surg. 2013 Dec;48(12):2408-15. https://doi.org/10.1016/j.jpedsurg.2013.08.014.)

Mesh closure

There are numerous materials available for a mesh-based patch closure. The most common is polytetrafluoroethylene (PTFE), a synthetic polymer. The most common biologic mesh used is small intestinal submucosa (SIS). Most surgeons now favor synthetic polymers such as PTFE to reduce recurrence risk, which has been validated in recent small studies.[81–83] When a mesh-based closure is chosen several tenants must be kept in mind.

- A subcostal incision on the side of the hernia is then made approximately one finger breath or less below the costal margin with extension both laterally and medially to perform the procedure (see **Fig. 1**). The location of this incision relative to the costal margin balances the ability to easily visualize the hernia defect with the ability to close the abdominal wall on completion of the procedure.

- Laxity or "doming" of the mesh is recommended. This dome allows the child to grow without creating undo stress on the interface between the mesh and the natural diaphragmatic tissues.
- Like most muscular hernias, there should be a considerable overlap between native diaphragm and the mesh to promote strength when possible. Most surgeons will approximate the muscular diaphragm to mesh closure using a horizontal-type mattress suture (with or without pledges) with minimal spacing in between each mattress suture (**Fig. 3**).
- In the scenario where there is no native diaphragm, pericostal mattress sutures can be used to recreate the diaphragm with the mesh.
- In large type C and type D defects, closing the medial space around the great vessels and

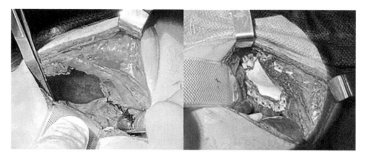

Fig. 3. Mesh-based closure of a right-sided CDH. (*Left*) Note the primary closure of the medial aspect of the defect. (*Right*) PTFE-based mesh closure with buttress using a horizontal mattress pattern and nonabsorbable suture. (Photo courtesy of Irving J. Zamora, M.D.)

the esophagus is difficult and requires creativity regarding to structure a closure that prevents additional herniation while avoiding angulation of traversing structures. In the setting of limited tissue, priority should be given to close the medial side of the defect. A known complication of CDH with medial defects is para-esophageal hernias.

Myofascial flap

There have been several techniques described using a portion of the abdominal wall musculature on the ipsilateral side of the defect to provide coverage.[84,85] At our institution, we have used a flap containing the transversalis fascia/muscle that extends to include the posterior sheath of the rectus abdominis medially (see **Fig. 1**).

- The surgery is started by creating a transverse incision on the abdominal wall that is approximately a finger breadth above to the umbilicus and extends just medial to the costal border on the affected side (see **Fig. 1**).
- The abdominal wall musculature is then opened, and the hernia contents are reduced. Once it is determined that the hernia is not amenable to primary repair, the transversalis muscle as well as the fascia is mobilized with blunt dissection and electrocautery away from the internal oblique. The fascia between the transversalis muscle and the internal oblique is dissected so that it stays with the myofascial flap.
- Dissection is then extended medially onto the rectus muscle all the way to the linea alba.

Importantly, the posterior sheath is maintained with the flap. Once the linea alba is reached, the flap is divided in the super direction extending superiorly up to the costal margin if needed facilitating a broad range of coverage depending on the size of the defect. The inferomedial aspect of the flap will cover the posteromedial component of the hernia defect. The defect is then covered/closed. Finally, the abdominal wall musculature is closed in one layer.

Thoracoscopy

Thoracoscopic repair of CDH is somewhat controversial given multiple reports of higher rates of recurrence.[86–89] Proponents of thoracoscopic repair cite reduced postoperative bowel obstructions along with traditional benefits of minimally invasive surgery. Thoracoscopy is generally reserved for low-risk patients with smaller (ie, Type A/B) defects that will likely be amenable to primary closure, but synthetic mesh can be placed thoracoscopically.[90] Thoracoscopic approach is initiated after general anesthesia by placing the patient sideways on the operative table with monitors at the patient's feet. The patient is then placed in a steep lateral decubitus position (ie, almost prone) with the affected side up (**Fig. 4**).

- Initial trocar placement (3/4 mm) is in the third or fourth intercostal space anterior to the tip of the scapula after insufflating the affected side with carbon dioxide via a Veress needle to 3 to 5 mm Hg. This is typically well tolerated in the low-risk patient.

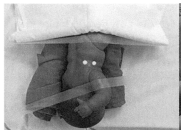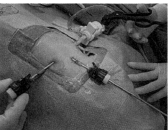

Fig. 4. VATS CDH Repair. (*Left*) General positioning of the patient with the red circle denoting position the camera port and the yellow circles denoting the working ports. (*Right*) Operative photo of the same trocar positioning. (Photo courtesy of Irving J. Zamora, M.D.)

- Additional 3 to 5 mm trocars are then placed as working ports one to two rib spaces below and camera right/camera left of the initial trocar. Appropriate triangulation of these two trocars is imperative for ease of operation. Similarly, the patient's arm on the affected side may impede the ports and must be kept in mind during positioning/padding.
- The initial steps of the operation involve reduction of hollow viscera first and then the solid organs. In a left-sided CDH, care must be taken to not injure the spleen; this is reduced last and functions as a "cap" for closure of the defect. The size and exact location of the hernia defect is then assessed.
- If there is a posterior muscular ring any retroperitoneal attachments are dissected free.
- The ability to close the defect primarily is assessed.
- If amenable to primary repair, the investigators typically use a biologic (SIS) underlay mesh to theoretically reduce the risk of recurrence.[91] This is completed configuring the mesh with a 1-cm underlay circumferentially. The edges of the hernia defect are scored with electrocautery to promote scarring.
- The mesh is then rolled tightly and introduced into the chest through one of the trocar sites. The proposed site for the second most medial suture is then completed first. The mesh is then unrolled and delivered under the defect using an absorbable suture in the mesh to aid placement. The most medial stitch is then placed and incorporates a bite of both muscular leaflets and a small component of the mesh (**Fig. 5**).
- The diaphragm is then closed in interrupted type fashion with nonabsorbable suture incorporating the mesh, typically in a medial to lateral approach. The authors typically use 2-0 or 3-0 silk suture thoracoscopically.
- Like the open technique, when the lateral margin of the hernia does not include diaphragm, pericostal sutures must be used. In the thoracoscopic approach, this can be completed with a stab incision externally overlying the rib that will be used for fixation.

The suture needle is then passed externally to internally through this site, securing the tail with a snap. The needle is passed inferior to the rib, the diaphragm is incorporated in the next bite, and finally the needle is then passed superiorly to the rib and out through the same stab incision and tied (see **Fig. 5**).
- When the defect is not amenable to primary closure, the surgeon can choose to convert to laparotomy or place synthetic mesh thoracoscopically. Synthetic mesh placement thoracoscopically is technically challenging and controversial, given the reported higher rates of recurrence associated with both the technique and larger defects.

SURGICAL COMPLICATIONS

The most common postoperative complications related to CDH repair are hernia recurrence and bowel obstruction. Children with CDH are also prone to developing gastroesophageal reflux, which requires surveillance, occasionally medical therapy, and surgery in severe/refractory cases.[6,92] Any child with significant/refractory gastroesophageal reflux and a history of CDH should be evaluated for hernia recurrence.

Hernia Recurrence

The clinical presentation for a CDH recurrence is highly variable. Although a large proportion of recurrences will be found in asymptomatic patients on screening chest x-ray, some may present with respiratory distress or signs of bowel obstruction. The rate of hernia recurrence is partially based on the size of the initial defect, the surgical approach, and the nature of the closure. Thoracoscopic repair has also been reported to have a higher recurrence rate even when controlling for defect size and other comorbidities.[89,93] Thoracoscopic repair confers a lower risk for postoperative bowel obstruction, but this must be weighed against hernia recurrence and is surgeon-dependent.[90,93,94]

The general rate of recurrence is typically quoted at 6% to 12% for open repair.[6,92,95] Larger defects, such as those with liver up and/or requiring patch repair, have historically reported

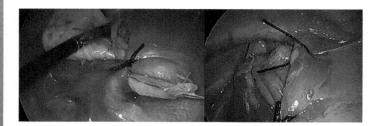

Fig. 5. VATS CDH hernia closure. (*Left*) Placement of initial closing suture and delivering SIS mesh under the defect. (*Right*) Lateral peri-costal suture placement. (Photos courtesy of Irving J. Zamora, M.D.)

recurrence rates as high as 50%.[6,95,96] Most of the recurrences occur within the first year of repair and decline significantly after the third year of life.[6,94,96,97] Surveillance through this time period is necessary, and some clinicians monitor annually until adolescence.[6,94,96,97]

Creating a dome in the mesh to produce a redundant/tension-free repair reportedly reduces hernia recurrence.[98,99] Aydin and colleagues recently reported equal recurrence rates and time to recurrence in mesh versus myofascial closure, and Dewberry and colleagues reported a lower recurrence rate with myofascial closure in a similar cohort of patients.[84,97]

Small Bowel Obstruction

Small bowel obstruction (SBO) after CDH repair is most commonly due to adhesive disease, followed by hernia recurrence and volvulus.[94,100] Reported rates for SBO are 6% to 20%, depending on the approach and use of mesh. Laparotomy and mesh utilization confer higher rates of SBO in most studies.[6,92,94,95]

SUMMARY

CHD is benefitted by a multidisciplinary approach in a high-volume center to achieve optimal outcomes. Additional studies and data will be useful to better select timing and method of repair on an individual basis.

CLINICS CARE POINTS

- Optimal medical care for neonates with CDH should be based upon national/international guidelines and delivered by multidisciplinary teams with experience in this patient population.
- Timing of surgical repair is based upon physiologic status and need for ECMO.

DISCLOSURE

The authors have nothing to disclose.

REFERENCES

1. Doyle NM, Lally KP. The CDH Study Group and advances in the clinical care of the patient with congenital diaphragmatic hernia. Semin Perinatol 2004;28(3):174–84.
2. Wynn J, Krishnan U, Aspelund G, et al. Outcomes of congenital diaphragmatic hernia in the modern era of management. J Pediatr 2013;163(1):114–119 e1.
3. Wynn J, Yu L, Chung WK. Genetic causes of congenital diaphragmatic hernia. Semin Fetal Neonatal Med 2014;19(6):324–30.
4. Harrison MR, Bjordal RI, Langmark F, et al. Congenital diaphragmatic hernia: the hidden mortality. J Pediatr Surg 1978;13(3):227–30.
5. Garcia A, Stolar CJ. Congenital diaphragmatic hernia and protective ventilation strategies in pediatric surgery. Surg Clin North Am 2012;92(3):659–68, ix.
6. Zani A, Chung WK, Deprest J, et al. Congenital diaphragmatic hernia. Nat Rev Dis Primers 2022;8(1):37.
7. Harting MT, Lally KP. The Congenital Diaphragmatic Hernia Study Group registry update. Semin Fetal Neonatal Med 2014;19(6):370–5.
8. Holder AM, Klaassens M, Tibboel D, et al. Genetic factors in congenital diaphragmatic hernia. Am J Hum Genet 2007;80(5):825–45.
9. Bargy F, Beaudoin S, Barbet P. Fetal lung growth in congenital diaphragmatic hernia. Fetal Diagn Ther 2006;21(1):39–44.
10. Byrne FA, Keller RL, Meadows J, et al. Severe left diaphragmatic hernia limits size of fetal left heart more than does right diaphragmatic hernia. Ultrasound Obstet Gynecol 2015;46(6):688–94.
11. Kitagawa M, Hislop A, Boyden EA, et al. Lung hypoplasia in congenital diaphragmatic hernia. A quantitative study of airway, artery, and alveolar development. Br J Surg 1971;58(5):342–6.
12. De Leon N, Tse WH, Ameis D, et al. Embryology and anatomy of congenital diaphragmatic hernia. Semin Pediatr Surg 2022;31(6):151229.
13. Gupta VS, Harting MT. Congenital diaphragmatic hernia-associated pulmonary hypertension. Semin Perinatol 2020;44(1):151167.
14. Cordier AG, Russo FM, Deprest J, et al. Prenatal diagnosis, imaging, and prognosis in Congenital Diaphragmatic Hernia. Semin Perinatol 2020;44(1):51163.
15. Raitio A, Salim A, Losty PD. Congenital diaphragmatic hernia-does the presence of a hernia sac improve outcome? A systematic review of published studies. Eur J Pediatr 2021;180(2):333–7.
16. Menon SC, Tani LY, Weng HY, et al. Clinical characteristics and outcomes of patients with cardiac defects and congenital diaphragmatic hernia. J Pediatr 2013;162(1):114–119 e2.
17. Oh T, Chan S, Kieffer S, et al. Fetal Outcomes of Prenatally Diagnosed Congenital Diaphragmatic Hernia: Nine Years of Clinical Experience in a Canadian Tertiary Hospital. J Obstet Gynaecol Can 2016;38(1):17–22.
18. Ba'ath ME, Jesudason EC, Losty PD. How useful is the lung-to-head ratio in predicting outcome in the fetus with congenital diaphragmatic hernia? A

systematic review and meta-analysis. Ultrasound Obstet Gynecol 2007;30(6):897–906.

19. Gallot D, Boda C, Ughetto S, et al. Prenatal detection and outcome of congenital diaphragmatic hernia: a French registry-based study. Ultrasound Obstet Gynecol 2007;29(3):276–83.

20. Jancelewicz T, Brindle ME. Prediction tools in congenital diaphragmatic hernia. Semin Perinatol 2020;44(1):151165.

21. Metkus AP, Filly RA, Stringer MD, et al. Sonographic predictors of survival in fetal diaphragmatic hernia. J Pediatr Surg 1996;31(1):148–51 [discussion 151-2].

22. Deprest JA, Flemmer AW, Gratacos E, et al. Antenatal prediction of lung volume and in-utero treatment by fetal endoscopic tracheal occlusion in severe isolated congenital diaphragmatic hernia. Semin Fetal Neonatal Med 2009;14(1):8–13.

23. Deprest JA, Nicolaides KH, Benachi A, et al. Randomized Trial of Fetal Surgery for Severe Left Diaphragmatic Hernia. N Engl J Med 2021;385(2):107–18.

24. Perrone EE, Abbasi N, Cortes MS, et al. Prenatal assessment of congenital diaphragmatic hernia at north american fetal therapy network centers: A continued plea for standardization. Prenat Diagn 2021;41(2):200–6.

25. Victoria T, Danzer E, Adzick NS. Use of ultrasound and MRI for evaluation of lung volumes in fetuses with isolated left congenital diaphragmatic hernia. Semin Pediatr Surg 2013;22(1):30–6.

26. Sperling JD, Sparks TN, Berger VK, et al. Prenatal Diagnosis of Congenital Diaphragmatic Hernia: Does Laterality Predict Perinatal Outcomes? Am J Perinatol 2018;35(10):919–24.

27. DeKoninck P, Gomez O, Sandaite I, et al. Right-sided congenital diaphragmatic hernia in a decade of fetal surgery. BJOG 2015;122(7):940–6.

28. Harrison MR, Keller RL, Hawgood SB, et al. A randomized trial of fetal endoscopic tracheal occlusion for severe fetal congenital diaphragmatic hernia. N Engl J Med 2003;349(20):1916–24.

29. Deprest JA, Benachi A, Gratacos E, et al. Randomized Trial of Fetal Surgery for Moderate Left Diaphragmatic Hernia. N Engl J Med 2021;385(2):119–29.

30. Morche J, Mathes T, Jacobs A, et al. Relationship between volume and outcome for surgery on congenital diaphragmatic hernia: A systematic review. J Pediatr Surg 2020;55(12):2555–65.

31. Badillo A, Gingalewski C. Congenital diaphragmatic hernia: treatment and outcomes. Semin Perinatol 2014;38(2):92–6.

32. Canadian Congenital Diaphragmatic Hernia C, Puligandla PS, Skarsgard ED, et al. Diagnosis and management of congenital diaphragmatic hernia: a clinical practice guideline. CMAJ (Can Med Assoc J) 2018;190(4):E103–12.

33. Duncan KV, Polites S, Krishnaswami S, et al. Congenital Diaphragmatic Hernia Management: A Systematic Review and Care Pathway Description Including Volume-Targeted Ventilation. Adv Neonatal Care 2021;21(5):E138–43.

34. Guner Y, Jancelewicz T, Di Nardo M, et al. Management of Congenital Diaphragmatic Hernia Treated With Extracorporeal Life Support: Interim Guidelines Consensus Statement From the Extracorporeal Life Support Organization. ASAIO J 2021;67(2):113–20.

35. Jancelewicz T, Brindle ME, Guner YS, et al. Toward Standardized Management of Congenital Diaphragmatic Hernia: An Analysis of Practice Guidelines. J Surg Res 2019;243:229–35.

36. Snoek KG, Reiss IK, Greenough A, et al. Standardized Postnatal Management of Infants with Congenital Diaphragmatic Hernia in Europe: The CDH EURO Consortium Consensus - 2015 Update. Neonatology 2016;110(1):66–74.

37. Storme L, Boubnova J, Mur S, et al. Review shows that implementing a nationwide protocol for congenital diaphragmatic hernia was a key factor in reducing mortality and morbidity. Acta Paediatr 2018;107(7):1131–9.

38. Mimura K, Endo M, Kawanishi Y, et al. Neonatal outcomes of congenital diaphragmatic hernia in full term versus early term deliveries: A systematic review and meta-analysis. Prenat Diagn 2023;43(8):993–1001.

39. Cochius-den Otter SCM, Horn-Oudshoorn EJJ, Allegaert K, et al. Routine Intubation in Newborns With Congenital Diaphragmatic Hernia. Pediatrics 2020;146(4).

40. Sur A, Awoseliya A, Sharma A. Outcome Analysis of Congenital Diaphragmatic Hernia Cohort before and after Implementation of Standardized Protocol in a Tertiary Neonatal Unit. Surg J 2017;3(3):e139–42.

41. Patel N, Lally PA, Kipfmueller F, et al. Ventricular Dysfunction Is a Critical Determinant of Mortality in Congenital Diaphragmatic Hernia. Am J Respir Crit Care Med 2019;200(12):1522–30.

42. Patel N, Massolo AC, Kipfmueller F. Congenital diaphragmatic hernia-associated cardiac dysfunction. Semin Perinatol 2020;44(1):151168.

43. Yang MJ, Russell KW, Yoder BA, et al. Congenital diaphragmatic hernia: a narrative review of controversies in neonatal management. Transl Pediatr 2021;10(5):1432–47.

44. Riley JS, Antiel RM, Rintoul NE, et al. Reduced oxygen concentration for the resuscitation of infants with congenital diaphragmatic hernia. J Perinatol 2018;38(7):834–43.

45. Yang MJ, Fenton S, Russell K, et al. Left-sided congenital diaphragmatic hernia: can we improve

survival while decreasing ECMO? J Perinatol 2020; 40(6):935–42.

46. Williams E, Greenough A. Respiratory Support of Infants With Congenital Diaphragmatic Hernia. Front Pediatr 2021;9:808317.

47. Snoek KG, Capolupo I, van Rosmalen J, et al. Conventional Mechanical Ventilation Versus High-frequency Oscillatory Ventilation for Congenital Diaphragmatic Hernia: A Randomized Clinical Trial (The VICI-trial). Ann Surg 2016; 263(5):867–74.

48. Pierro M, Thebaud B. Understanding and treating pulmonary hypertension in congenital diaphragmatic hernia. Semin Fetal Neonatal Med 2014; 19(6):357–63.

49. Inhaled nitric oxide and hypoxic respiratory failure in infants with congenital diaphragmatic hernia. The Neonatal Inhaled Nitric Oxide Study Group (NINOS). Pediatrics 1997;99(6):838–45.

50. Campbell BT, Herbst KW, Briden KE, et al. Inhaled nitric oxide use in neonates with congenital diaphragmatic hernia. Pediatrics 2014;134(2): e420–6.

51. Putnam LR, Tsao K, Morini F, et al. Evaluation of Variability in Inhaled Nitric Oxide Use and Pulmonary Hypertension in Patients With Congenital Diaphragmatic Hernia. JAMA Pediatr 2016;170(12): 1188–94.

52. Noh CY, Chock VY, Bhombal S, et al. Early nitric oxide is not associated with improved outcomes in congenital diaphragmatic hernia. Pediatr Res 2023;93(7):1899–906.

53. Kipfmueller F, Schroeder L, Berg C, et al. Continuous intravenous sildenafil as an early treatment in neonates with congenital diaphragmatic hernia. Pediatr Pulmonol 2018;53(4):452–60.

54. Cochius-den Otter S, Schaible T, Greenough A, et al. The CoDiNOS trial protocol: an international randomised controlled trial of intravenous sildenafil versus inhaled nitric oxide for the treatment of pulmonary hypertension in neonates with congenital diaphragmatic hernia. BMJ Open 2019;9(11): e032122.

55. Hari Gopal S, Patel N, Fernandes CJ. Use of Prostaglandin E1 in the Management of Congenital Diaphragmatic Hernia-A Review. Front Pediatr 2022; 10:911588.

56. Vogel M, McElhinney DB, Marcus E, et al. Significance and outcome of left heart hypoplasia in fetal congenital diaphragmatic hernia. Ultrasound Obstet Gynecol 2010;35(3):310–7.

57. Acker SN, Kinsella JP, Abman SH, et al. Vasopressin improves hemodynamic status in infants with congenital diaphragmatic hernia. J Pediatr 2014;165(1):53–58 e1.

58. Capolupo I, De Rose DU, Mazzeo F, et al. Early vasopressin infusion improves oxygenation in infants with congenital diaphragmatic hernia. Front Pediatr 2023;11:1104728.

59. Rafat N, Schaible T. Extracorporeal Membrane Oxygenation in Congenital Diaphragmatic Hernia. Front Pediatr 2019;7:336.

60. Barbaro RP, Paden ML, Guner YS, et al. Pediatric Extracorporeal Life Support Organization Registry International Report 2016. ASAIO J 2017;63(4): 456–63.

61. Cairo SB, Arbuthnot M, Boomer LA, et al. Controversies in extracorporeal membrane oxygenation (ECMO) utilization and congenital diaphragmatic hernia (CDH) repair using a Delphi approach: from the American Pediatric Surgical Association Critical Care Committee (APSA-CCC). Pediatr Surg Int 2018;34(11):1163–9.

62. Delaplain PT, Jancelewicz T, Di Nardo M, et al. Management preferences in ECMO mode for congenital diaphragmatic hernia. J Pediatr Surg 2019;54(5):903–8.

63. Cho HJ, Kim DW, Kim GS, et al. Anticoagulation Therapy during Extracorporeal Membrane Oxygenator Support in Pediatric Patients. Chonnam Med J 2017;53(2):110–7.

64. Kim AG, Mon R, Karmakar M, et al. Predicting lethal pulmonary hypoplasia in congenital diaphragmatic hernia (CDH): Institutional experience combined with CDH registry outcomes. J Pediatr Surg 2020;55(12):2618–24.

65. Kays DW, Islam S, Richards DS, et al. Extracorporeal life support in patients with congenital diaphragmatic hernia: how long should we treat? J Am Coll Surg. Apr 2014;218(4):808–17.

66. Harting MT, Jancelewicz T. Surgical Management of Congenital Diaphragmatic Hernia. Clin Perinatol 2022;49(4):893–906.

67. Hollinger LE, Lally PA, Tsao K, et al. A risk-stratified analysis of delayed congenital diaphragmatic hernia repair: does timing of operation matter? Surgery 2014;156(2):475–82.

68. Gentili A, Pasini L, Iannella E, et al. Predictive outcome indexes in neonatal Congenital Diaphragmatic Hernia. J Matern Fetal Neonatal Med 2015; 28(13):1602–7.

69. Logan JW, Rice HE, Goldberg RN, et al. Congenital diaphragmatic hernia: a systematic review and summary of best-evidence practice strategies. J Perinatol. Sep 2007;27(9):535–49.

70. Snyder CW, Goldenberg NA, Nguyen ATH, et al. A perioperative bivalirudin anticoagulation protocol for neonates with congenital diaphragmatic hernia on extracorporeal membrane oxygenation. Thromb Res. Sep 2020;193:198–203.

71. Kaushik S, Derespina KR, Chandhoke S, et al. Use of bivalirudin for anticoagulation in pediatric extracorporeal membrane oxygenation (ECMO). Perfusion. Jan 2023;38(1):58–65.

72. Ryerson LM, Balutis KR, Granoski DA, et al. Prospective Exploratory Experience With Bivalirudin Anticoagulation in Pediatric Extracorporeal Membrane Oxygenation. Pediatr Crit Care Med. Nov 2020;21(11):975–85.

73. Ryerson LM, McMichael ABV. Bivalirudin in pediatric extracorporeal membrane oxygenation. Curr Opin Pediatr 2022;34(3):255–60.

74. Seelhammer TG, Bohman JK, Schulte PJ, et al. Comparison of Bivalirudin Versus Heparin for Maintenance Systemic Anticoagulation During Adult and Pediatric Extracorporeal Membrane Oxygenation. Crit Care Med 2021;49(9):1481–92.

75. Valdes CA, Sharaf OM, Bleiweis MS, et al. Heparin-based versus bivalirudin-based anticoagulation in pediatric extracorporeal membrane oxygenation: A systematic review. Front Med 2023;10:1137134.

76. Congenital Diaphragmatic Hernia Study G, Bryner BS, West BT, et al. Congenital diaphragmatic hernia requiring extracorporeal membrane oxygenation: does timing of repair matter? J Pediatr Surg 2009;44(6):1165–71 [discussion 1171-2].

77. Partridge EA, Peranteau WH, Rintoul NE, et al. Timing of repair of congenital diaphragmatic hernia in patients supported by extracorporeal membrane oxygenation (ECMO). J Pediatr Surg. Feb 2015; 50(2):260–2.

78. Dao DT, Burgos CM, Harting MT, et al. Surgical Repair of Congenital Diaphragmatic Hernia After Extracorporeal Membrane Oxygenation Cannulation: Early Repair Improves Survival. Ann Surg 2021;274(1):186–94.

79. Dassinger MS, Copeland DR, Gossett J, et al. Early repair of congenital diaphragmatic hernia on extracorporeal membrane oxygenation. J Pediatr Surg. Apr 2010;45(4):693–7.

80. Lally KP, Lasky RE, Lally PA, et al. Standardized reporting for congenital diaphragmatic hernia–an international consensus. J Pediatr Surg 2013; 48(12):2408–15.

81. de Haro Jorge I, Prat Ortells J, Martin-Sole O, et al. Porcine dermal patches as a risk factor for recurrence after congenital diaphragmatic hernia repair. Pediatr Surg Int. Jan 2021;37(1):59–65.

82. Ruhrnschopf CG, Reusmann A, Boglione M, et al. Biological versus synthetic patch for the repair of congenital diaphragmatic hernia: 8-year experience at a tertiary center. J Pediatr Surg. Nov 2021;56(11):1957–61.

83. Schlager A, Arps K, Siddharthan R, et al. Tube Thoracostomy at the Time of Congenital Diaphragmatic Hernia Repair: Reassessing the Risks and Benefits. J Laparoendosc Adv Surg Tech A. Mar 2017;27(3):311–7.

84. Dewberry L, Hilton S, Gien J, et al. Flap repair in congenital diaphragmatic hernia leads to lower rates of recurrence. J Pediatr Surg 2019;54(12): 2487–91.

85. Scaife ER, Johnson DG, Meyers RL, et al. The split abdominal wall muscle flap–a simple, mesh-free approach to repair large diaphragmatic hernia. J Pediatr Surg 2003;38(12):1748–51.

86. Clifton MS and Wulkan ML. Thoracoscopic congenital diaphragmatic hernia repair, In: Holcomb GW III, Rothenberg SS, editors. Atlas of pediatric laparoscopy and thoracoscopy, 2nd edition, 2022, Elsevier. 247-251.

87. Rideout DA, Wulkan M. Thoracoscopic Neonatal Congenital Diaphragmatic Hernia Repair: How We Do It. J Laparoendosc Adv Surg Tech 2021; 31(10):1168–74.

88. Arca MJ, Barnhart DC, Lelli JL Jr, et al. Early experience with minimally invasive repair of congenital diaphragmatic hernias: results and lessons learned. J Pediatr Surg 2003;38(11):1563–8.

89. Putnam LR, Gupta V, Tsao K, et al. Factors associated with early recurrence after congenital diaphragmatic hernia repair. J Pediatr Surg 2017; 52(6):928–32.

90. Lacher M, St Peter SD, Laje P, et al. Thoracoscopic CDH Repair–A Survey on Opinion and Experience Among IPEG Members. J Laparoendosc Adv Surg Tech A 2015;25(11):954–7.

91. Vandewalle RJ, Yalcin S, Clifton MS, et al. Biologic Mesh Underlay in Thoracoscopic Primary Repair of Congenital Diaphragmatic Hernia Confers Reduced Recurrence in Neonates: A Preliminary Report. J Laparoendosc Adv Surg Tech 2019; 29(10):1212–5.

92. Yokota K, Uchida H, Kaneko K, et al. Surgical complications, especially gastroesophageal reflux disease, intestinal adhesion obstruction, and diaphragmatic hernia recurrence, are major sequelae in survivors of congenital diaphragmatic hernia. Pediatr Surg Int 2014;30(9):895–9.

93. Putnam LR, Tsao K, Lally KP, et al. Minimally Invasive vs Open Congenital Diaphragmatic Hernia Repair: Is There a Superior Approach? J Am Coll Surg 2017;224(4):416–22.

94. Zahn KB, Franz AM, Schaible T, et al. Small Bowel Obstruction After Neonatal Repair of Congenital Diaphragmatic Hernia-Incidence and Risk-Factors Identified in a Large Longitudinal Cohort-Study. Front Pediatr 2022;10:846630.

95. Heiwegen K, de Blaauw I, Botden S. A systematic review and meta-analysis of surgical morbidity of primary versus patch repaired congenital diaphragmatic hernia patients. Sci Rep 2021;11(1): 12661.

96. Moss RL, Chen CM, Harrison MR. Prosthetic patch durability in congenital diaphragmatic hernia: a long-term follow-up study. J Pediatr Surg. Jan 2001;36(1):152–4.

97. Aydin E, Nolan H, Peiro JL, et al. When primary repair is not enough: a comparison of synthetic patch and muscle flap closure in congenital diaphragmatic hernia? Pediatr Surg Int 2020;36(4):485–91.

98. Suply E, Rees C, Cross K, et al. Patch repair of congenital diaphragmatic hernia is not at risk of poor outcomes. J Pediatr Surg 2020;55(8): 1522–7.

99. Verla MA, Style CC, Lee TC, et al. Does creating a dome reduce recurrence in congenital diaphragmatic hernia following patch repair? J Pediatr Surg 2022;57(4):637–42.

100. Jancelewicz T, Vu LT, Keller RL, et al. Long-term surgical outcomes in congenital diaphragmatic hernia: observations from a single institution. J Pediatr Surg 2010;45(1):155–60 [discussion 160].

Management of Congenital Hernias in Adults: Foramen of Morgagni Hernia

Nicolas Contreras, MD[a,b], Thomas K. Varghese Jr, MD, MS, MBA[a,b],
Brian Mitzman, MD, MS[a,b],*

KEYWORDS

• Morgagni hernia • Diaphragm • Surgery • Robotic

KEY POINTS

- Morgagni hernias are defects in the anterior diaphragm due to a malformation in the fibrotendinous elements that fuse behind the sternum.
- Most patients are asymptomatic, but symptoms can be severe based on the size of the defect and the contents of the hernia.
- Repairs are often completed successfully using a laparoscopic approach despite large hernia contents, but alternative approaches may be necessary in complex clinical situations.
- Mesh is rarely needed when transfascial repair sutures are utilized, but may be required for larger defects.

INTRODUCTION

The Morgagni hernia, a defect named after the famed Italian anatomist Giovanni Battista Morgagni, occurs through the sternocostal triangle. Although the Morgagni hernia itself will be the focus of this review, one does not simply gloss over Morgagni's name without paying a few lines of special tribute to a giant in the history of medicine, and someone who is considered the father of modern Anatomic Pathology.[1,2] Born in Italy in 1682, Morgagni had an illustrious 56-year career as a professor of anatomy at the prestigious University of Padua. His career was flanked by other giants in the history of medicine—he was the pupil of Antonio Valsalva and the professor to Antonio Scarpa. Prior to Morgagni, normal human anatomy had been exhaustively described; however, a systematic description of anatomy with a focus on diseased organs had never been performed, which is Morgagni's most notable legacy. In 1761, Morgagni published his greatest work, *De Sedibus et Causis Morborum per Anatomen Indagatis (The Seats and Causes of Diseases Investigated by Anatomy)*, containing records of 640 different dissections. In it, he highlighted the importance of diagnosis, prognosis, and treatment on a comprehensive knowledge of anatomic conditions.[3,4] Eponymous structures from the sinuses of the pharynx to the columnar folds of the anal canal bare Morgagni's name, including the foramen of Morgagni (sternocostal triangle) through which Morgagni hernias occur. Given the special tribute to Giovanni Morgagni, the authors first will begin the review with an anatomic description of the diaphragm and the anatomic defects leading to hernia pathology, followed by clinical presentation, evaluation, and current surgical treatments for Morgagni hernias, including robotic approaches to repair.

ANATOMY

The anatomic details pertinent to Morgagni hernias are reviewed herein, for more comprehensive details

Funding: None.
a Division of Cardiothoracic Surgery, Department of Surgery, University of Utah Health, 30 N Mario Capechi Drive, Salt Lake City, UT, USA; b Huntsman Cancer Institute, 1950 Circle of Hope, Salt Lake City, UT, USA
* Corresponding author. Huntsman Cancer Hospital (North), 1950 Circle of Hope, Office K7526, Salt Lake City, UT 84112.
E-mail address: brian.mitzman@hsc.utah.edu

Thorac Surg Clin 34 (2024) 147–154
https://doi.org/10.1016/j.thorsurg.2024.01.004
1547-4127/24/© 2024 Elsevier Inc. All rights reserved.

regarding diaphragmatic anatomy, please refer to Chapter 1. The sternocostal triangle, or Foramen of Morgagni, is a space behind the sternum in between the lateral edge of the diaphragm and the sternocostal attachments where a defect may form due to incomplete fusion of the septum transversum and the sternum.[5] This failure of fusion of the fibrotendinous elements often leads to a right-sided hernia (90% of Morgagni hernia patients) due to pericardial attachments on the left preventing herniation.[6] A left- sided sternocostal triangle hernia is often referred to as a Larrey Hernia.[7] This eponym is given from Napoleon's famed war surgeon, Dominque-Jean Larrey, who described a surgical approach to the pericardial cavity through a left anterior diaphragmatic defect.[8] Overall, Morgagni hernia makes up less than 3% of all congenital diaphragmatic hernias.[9] These hernias are generally not associated with other malformations or hernias in adults, and many are asymptomatic. Morgagni famously wrote:

> ...whenever the stomach is carried up through the diaphragm into the thorax...it does not always happen through a passage open'd by a wounding instrument...thus also, anteriorly, betwixt the fibres that come from the xyphoid cartilage and the neighbouring fibres, there generally is an interval through which something similar may happen: and I even suspect this to have happen'd in a husbandman in whom part of the intestine colon carried up through the middle and anterior part of the diaphragm...[10,11]

PRESENTATION

The presentation of a Morgagni hernia is varied, and depends on the size of hernia and contents protruding into the thorax.[6,12–14] The majority of patients are asymptomatic, presenting only after incidental discovery on chest X-ray or computed tomography (CT) scan performed for alternative reason.[15] These patients often have omentum or a small piece of non-incarcerated bowel protruding through the defect. When the hernia contains a larger portion of the intestine or stomach or a smaller/tighter defect, gastrointestinal symptoms may occur.[6,9,16,17] If a large portion of the hemithorax is compromised by hernia contents, respiratory complaints are common. Chest pain is a usual manifestation in those who are symptomatic, due to irritation of the epigastric plane.

EVALUATION AND TREATMENT

The clinical presentation and complexity of an operation will depend on the size of the hernia defect and the contents protruding into the mediastinum and thorax. To facilitate our discussion of the broad range of presentations and surgical management of Morgagni hernias, the authors have chosen 3 separate case scenarios with progressive degrees of complexity that will highlight some of the important nuances in surgical management.

Case 1—Simple Morgagni Hernia

A 68-year-old male presented with an incidental finding of Morgagni hernia after undergoing a chest X-ray during work up for a viral respiratory infection. A subsequent CT scan revealed an anterior fat-filled diaphragmatic hernia (**Fig. 1**). Initially surveilled due to pending recovery from his viral infection, the patient eventually developed intermittent epigastric pain which he attributed to the hernia. He subsequently opted to undergo repair.

In the modern era of surgical technique, a minimally invasive approach should be the standard option for repair—this may be either conventional laparoscopy or robotically assisted.[18–21] If utilizing a robotic approach with the da Vinci XI system (Intuitive Surgical; California), standard port placement for upper gastrointestinal laparoscopic surgery is utilized, with four 8-mm working ports. An accessory port for assistance and introduction of sutures is optional. **Fig. 2** shows intraoperative photos during repair of this simple fat-containing Morgagni hernia. Hernia contents are first identified (see **Fig. 2**A) and subsequently reduced to allow visualization of the anterior defect (see **Fig. 2**B). A liver retractor is not necessary, as the defect sits anterior to the liver. As with other diaphragmatic hernias, it is imperative to remove the entirety of the hernia sac from the defect prior to closure. These hernias are a direct failure of fusion between the diaphragm and posterior portion of the sternum. Therefore, there will not be any rim of diaphragm anteriorly for reconstruction. If small, as in this case, the diaphragm can be reapproximated to the sternum and costal cartilage. Braided non-absorbable polyester suture is utilized on felt pledgets and passed through the diaphragmatic edge in an interrupted mattress fashion. The sutures are brought through the fascia of the abdominal wall, the ends delivered through small 2 mm individual skin incisions and the sutures secured (see **Fig. 2**C). Critically, the diaphragm should not be under undue tension and complete closure achieved (see **Fig. 2**D).

A suture passer facilitates the placement of the transfascial stitches and many simple Morgagni hernia defects can be closed efficiently in this manner.

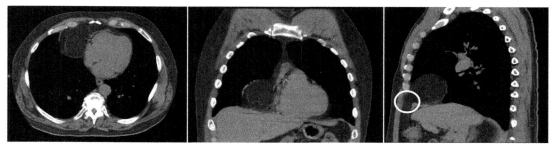

Fig. 1. CT imaging of simple right-sided fat-containing Morgagni hernia. White circle depicts anterior hernia defect.

This technique has been described throughout the literature with repeated success.[18,20–22]

The preoperative chest X-ray is shown in **Fig. 3**, with classic ovoid opacity just to the right of the sternum (3a), and the subsequent resolution after repair (3b).

Case 2—Difficult Morgagni Hernia

When significant portions of the abdominal viscera and contents protrude through a Morgagni hernia, patients may present with pain or gastrointestinal symptoms such as intermittent obstruction. The mobilization of larger, longer standing hernias increases some complexity along with a larger size of hernia; however, despite this, repair can often be performed in the same manner as a simple Morgagni hernia.

A 45-year-old female presented to the emergency room with progressive shortness of breath and dyspnea on exertion. She noted a history of epigastric pain which she contributed to gastrointestinal reflux disease. A CT chest was performed, which noted a large Morgagni diaphragmatic defect (**Fig. 4**A: axial, B: sagittal, C: Coronal). Hernia contents included abdominal fat and the transverse colon occupying the majority of the right hemithorax. There was also cranial displacement of her distal stomach due to the dispositioned colon. No volvulus or obstruction was seen.

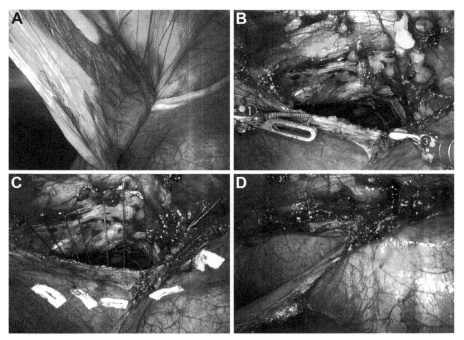

Fig. 2. Operative photos of simple Morgagni hernia. (*A*) Omentum protruding into mediastinum via hernia defect. (*B*) Hernia has been reduced, anterior defect visualized. (*C*) Transfascial mattress sutures placed with felt pledgets for repair. (*D*) Repaired hernia.

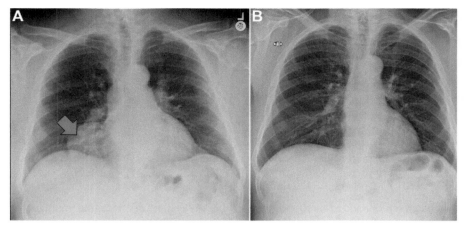

Fig. 3. Preoperative (*A*) and Postoperative (*B*) chest X-rays from repaired simple Morgagni hernia. Red arrow shows mediastinal hernia contents before repair.

Similar to the simple Morgagni repair, a minimally invasive approach should be attempted. By insufflating the abdomen, the defect routinely expands leading to easy reduction of the hernia contents. Reduced contents should be examined for injury and the hernia must be carefully examined to ensure completeness of reduction and resection of any hernia sac (**Fig. 5**A). Once reduced (**Fig. 5**B), a standard repair using transfascial buttressed sutures in a mattresses fashion can be utilized to reapproximate the diaphragm (**Fig. 5**C).

A Morgagni hernia with large volume of intra-abdominal contents can be misinterpreted for diaphragmatic elevation on chest X-ray alone. As seen in this patient's preoperative X-ray (**Fig. 6**A), it is difficult to interpret the location of abdominal contents without a lateral view of other more detailed imaging such as CT scan. A postoperative chest X-ray after reduction of abdominal contents and defect repair is also shown (**Fig. 6**B).

The primary repair of Morgagni hernias-containing bowel via laparoscopic approach has

been similarly described.[12,23] The method of repair is at the surgeon's discretion and should be determined based on size of the hernia defect and ability to reapproximate diaphragm directly to the anterior abdominal wall behind the sternum. If a primary repair results in undue tension or cannot be accomplished, use of mesh is appropriate. In some cases, a primary closure can be accomplished for the majority of the defect and mesh used to patch the remaining opening.[24–26] Like with a suture-repair, there is no anterior rim of diaphragm to which the mesh can be attached and transfascial sutures will be required for anterior anchoring of the patch.

Case 3—Convoluted Decision Making with a Gigantic Morgagni–Larrey Hernia

When a gigantic Morgagni hernia is combined with other urgent surgical problems, dilemmas may arise that require novel solutions.

A 63-year-old male with a history of Loeys–Dietz syndrome presented to the cardiac surgery

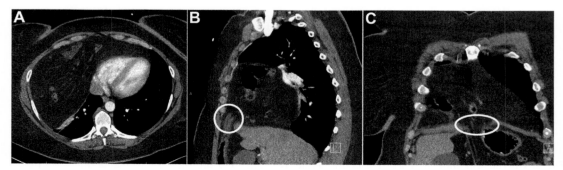

Fig. 4. CT imaging of complex right-sided Morgagni hernia containing omentum, small intestine, and large intestine. (*A*) Axial, (*B*) Sagittal, (*C*) Coronal. White circle depicts anterior hernia defect.

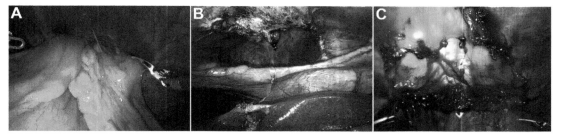

Fig. 5. Operative photos showing large complex Morgagni hernia containing intestine (*A*), reduced hernia with visualized anterior defect (*B*), and repaired hernia (*C*).

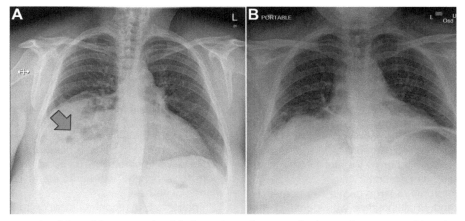

Fig. 6. Preoperative (*A*) and Postoperative (*B*) chest X-rays from repaired complex Morgagni hernia. Red arrow depicts right-sided hernia contents containing small and large intestines.

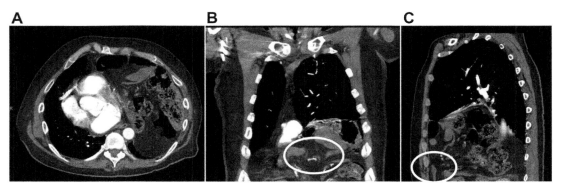

Fig. 7. CT imaging of gigantic complex left-sided Morgagni hernia containing small intestine, large intestine, and portion of the pancreas and spleen. (*A*) Axial, (*B*) Coronal, (*C*) Sagittal. White circle depicts a large anterior diaphragmatic defect.

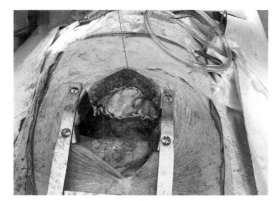

Fig. 8. Intraoperative photo showing repaired gigantic Morgagni–Larrey Hernia with Gore-Tex mesh via sternotomy. Head is oriented toward the bottom of the photo.

service with a bicuspid aortic valve and a dilated aortic root to 6.2 cm. This connective tissue disorder can often lead to recurrent hernias as well as arterial aneurysms. The patient had significant shortness of breath and unstable angina. On workup, he was found to have a gigantic Morgagni–Larrey hernia with the entirety of his transverse colon protruding into the left hemithorax (**Fig. 7**A: axial, B: coronal, C: sagittal). His cardiac surgery team determined that he needed urgent aortic root replacement, and the decision was made to fix his hernia via sternotomy at the time of his aortic operation.

After sternotomy, a large hernia sac containing both large and small intestine was identified protruding into the mediastinum and left hemithorax. This finding reinforces the dynamic and unpredictable nature of diaphragmatic hernias—imaging findings may change throughout the same hospitalization and differ from findings at the time of

surgical exploration. After reducing all the contacts with hernia sac back into the abdomen, the defect was measured and found to be 20 cm × 15 cm. This may have been partially due to stretching from the sternal retractor as there was substantial discordance with the preoperative imaging. Using a 2-mm thick Gore-Tex mesh, the defect was repaired with interrupted braided suture. Similar to laparoscopic repairs, the anterior rim of the defect was reapproximated to the abdominal wall by passing sutures transfascially and burying the knots beneath small skin incisions (**Fig. 8**). As described earlier, preoperative chest X-ray alone may misidentify large diaphragmatic hernias as an elevated hemidiaphragm (**Fig. 9**A). Postoperatively, chest X-ray and CT scan showed a completely reduced hernia with intact mesh (**Fig. 9**B and C).

When presented with non-standard scenarios, novel techniques must be utilized to facilitate safe repair. Hoyuela and colleagues described the use of cyanoacrylate glue for fixation of mesh to buttress primary repair in Morgagni hernias.[27] When presented with a combination of surgical issues, such as aortic disease and Morgagni hernia, multidisciplinary decision-making is essential in determining best course of care. Meng and colleagues describe the challenging decision-making in selecting order of procedures, approach of procedures, and detail a case of transcatheter aortic valve implantation to avoid the operating room for a patient with aortic stenosis and large Morgagni hernia.[28]

In patients with a contraindication to an abdominal approach, uncertain pathology, or the need for simultaneous chest surgery, video-assisted thoracoscopic or open trans-thoracic surgery may be utilized to repair anterior diaphragmatic hernias.[29,30]

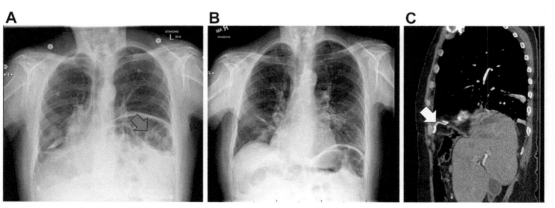

Fig. 9. Preoperative (*A*) and Postoperative (*B*) chest X-rays of gigantic complex left-sided Morgagni hernia. *Red arrow* depicts hernia. Sagittal CT scan after repair (*C*) with white arrow depicting Gore-Tex mesh repair of defect.

SUMMARY

Morgagni hernias are rare and often asymptomatic. They may be misinterpreted on standard chest X-ray, but are easily identifiable on CT scan. The standard approach in the modern era is laparoscopy, with or without robotic assistance. Often, primary repair can be accomplished utilizing transfascial sutures with excellent recurrence rates; however, mesh may be utilized in more complex scenarios.

CLINICS CARE POINTS

- When primarily reapproximating the diaphragm to the anterior abdominal wall, utilize interrupted sutures in a mattresses fashion with pledgets for longevity and strength.
- If unable to primarily repair the defect, a synthetic mesh such as 2-mm Gore-Tex should be used.
- While defects may be small, be prepared for large portions of the abdominal contents which may have herniated into the chest.

DISCLOSURE

B. Mitzman; Proctor for Intuitive Surgical.

REFERENCES

1. Ghosh SK. Giovanni Battista Morgagni (1682-1771): father of pathologic anatomy and pioneer of modern medicine. Anat Sci Int 2017;92(3):305–12.
2. Morgagni (1682-1771). JAMA 1964;187(12):948–50.
3. Adams EW. Founders of modern medicine: giovanni battista morgagni (1682-1771). Med Library Hist J 1903;1(4):270–7.
4. Hughes BD, Nakayama D. Giovanni battista morgagni and the morgagni hernia. Am Surg 2021. https://doi.org/10.1177/00031348211011108. 31348211011108.
5. Adereti C, Zahir J, Robinson E, et al. A Case Report and Literature Review on Incidental Morgagni Hernia in Bariatric Patients: To Repair or Not to Repair? Cureus 2023;15(6):e39950.
6. Modi M, Dey AK, Mate A, et al. Strangulated Morgagni's Hernia: A Rare Diagnosis and Management. Case Rep Surg 2016;2016:2621383.
7. Khan YA, ElKholy A. A missed complicated Morgagni–Larrey's hernia. Annals of Pediatric Surgery 2016;12(4):173–4.
8. Thomas TV. Subcostosternal diaphragmatic hernia. J Thorac Cardiovasc Surg 1972;63(2):279–83.
9. Young MC, Saddoughi SA, Aho JM, et al. Comparison of Laparoscopic Versus Open Surgical Management of Morgagni Hernia. Ann Thorac Surg 2019; 107(1):257–61.
10. Zani A, Cozzi DA. Giovanni battista morgagni and his contribution to pediatric surgery. J Pediatr Surg 2008;43(4):729–33.
11. Morgagni JB, ed. The Seats and Causes of Diseases Investigated by Anatomy (translated by B. Alexander). Millar, Cadell, Johnson and Payne; 1976. Morgagni JB, ed.
12. Albasheer O, Hakami N, Ahmed AA. Giant Morgagni hernia with transthoracic herniation of the left liver lobe and transverse colon: a case report. J Med Case Rep 2023;17(1):165.
13. Humble AG, Sample CB. Morgagni's hernia in a hypoxaemic adult. Lancet 2016;388(10045):705.
14. Huston JM, King H, Maresh A, et al. Hernia of Morgagni: case report. J Thorac Cardiovasc Surg 2008;135(1):212–3.
15. Svetanoff WJ, Rentea RM. Morgagni hernia. FL: StatPearls Publishing, Treasure Island; 2023.
16. Ben-Yaacov A, Menasherov N, Bard V. Repair of a recurrent symptomatic hernia through the foramen of Morgagni: a case study and review of the literature. J Surg Case Rep 2020;2020(7):rjaa230.
17. Marshall-Webb M, Thompson SK. Morgagni Hernia in an Adult: a Forgotten Cause of Epigastric Pain. J Gastrointest Surg 2023;27(3):628–30.
18. Hara T, Adachi T, Shimbara K, et al. Laparoscopic repair of Morgagni hernia with extra-abdominal sutures and ileocecal resection for colon cancer: a case report. J Surg Case Rep 2022;2022(12): rjac572.
19. Li J. Comment on: "Surgical technique in the laparoscopic repair of Morgagni hernia in adults. How do we do it?". Hernia 2022;26(6):1709–10.
20. Misra RP, Schwartz JD. A simplified technique of full-thickness transabdominal laparoscopic repair of Morgagni hernia. J Thorac Cardiovasc Surg 2011; 141(2):594–5.
21. Pulle MV, Asaf BB, Puri HV, et al. Robotic Morgagni's hernia repair in adults - A single centre experience. Asian Cardiovasc Thorac Ann 2023;31(3): 253–8.
22. Zaharie F, Valean D, Popa C, et al. Surgical technique in the laparoscopic repair of Morgagni hernia in adults. How do we do it? Hernia 2022;26(5): 1389–94.
23. Minneci PC, Deans KJ, Kim P, et al. Foramen of Morgagni hernia: changes in diagnosis and treatment. Ann Thorac Surg 2004;77(6):1956–9.
24. Rajkumar K, Kulkarni S, Talishinskiy T. Morgagni hernia: an uncommon pathology in adults. J Surg Case Rep 2022;2022(12):rjac597.

25. Stone ML, Julien MA, Dunnington GH Jr, et al. Novel laparoscopic hernia of Morgagni repair technique. J Thorac Cardiovasc Surg 2012;143(3):744–5.

26. Tzortzis AS, Papaconstantinou D. Letter to the Editor: Management of Morgagni's Hernia in the Adult Population: A Systematic Review of the Literature. World J Surg 2022;46(3):725–6.

27. Hoyuela C, Juvany M, Guillaumes S. Cyanoacrylate for Safer Mesh Fixation During Laparoscopic Repair of Morgagni Hernia. Ann Thorac Surg 2020;109(4):e305–7.

28. Meng E, Servito M, Alqaydi A, et al. Huge Morgagni Hernia, a Rare Criterion to Favor TAVI Against SAVR. JACC Case Rep 2023;11:101800.

29. Hussong RL Jr, Landreneau RJ, Cole FH Jr. Diagnosis and repair of a Morgagni hernia with video-assisted thoracic surgery. Ann Thorac Surg 1997; 63(5):1474–5.

30. Robinson BL, Shahian DM. Transthoracic repair of an unsuspected left foramen of Morgagni hernia. Ann Thorac Surg 2008;86(5):1693–5.

Congenital Hernias in Adults: Bochdalek Hernias

Connor J. Bridges, BS[a], Rian M. Hasson, MD, MPH[a,b,c],*

KEYWORDS

- Bochdalek hernias • Congenital hernias in adults • Management of Bochdalek hernias
- Surgical approach to Bochdalek hernias

KEY POINTS

- Bochdalek hernias are rare in adults but result from posterolateral defects of the diaphragm.
- Both symptomatic and asymptomatic Bochdalek hernias should be surgically repaired given the risk of acute mortality or morbidity.
- Surgical approach will depend on anatomy, acuity, and availability.

INTRODUCTION

Bochdalek hernias are a rare occurrence in adults. While many are discovered incidentally, some do present with symptoms secondary to the volume of herniated contents or potentially obstruction or strangulation of structures. Surgery is the mainstay of treatment. To begin, the authors share a recent case to help provide context to the diagnosis and treatment.

CASE

A 43-year-old man presented with 3 days of vomiting, abdominal pain, and a previous history significant for a hemorrhagic gastric ulcer 10 years prior. Following admission, a chest X-ray revealed nasogastric tube placement above the left diaphragm in addition to signs of bowel gas overlying the lung. A computed tomography (CT) scan revealed abdominal viscera herniated into the left thoracic cavity (**Fig. 1**). Ultimately, he was diagnosed with a left-sided Bochdalek hernia—a posterolateral diaphragmatic defect that, in this case, facilitated herniation of his stomach, pancreas, spleen, and colon into his chest. Surgical reduction of the hernia via L-shaped laparotomy proceeded without complication and the left lung was found to be fully expanded without any signs of pleural effusion or pulmonary edema on postoperative films (**Figs. 2 and 3**).[1]

BACKGROUND

Named after the work of Vincent Alexander Bochdalek, Bochdalek hernias have an estimated prevalence of 1 in 2200 to 1 in 12,500 live births.[2] They primarily present on the left side, which is suggested to be a result of later closure of the left diaphragmatic canal.[2] Several review articles have estimated right-sided Bochdalek hernias to account for only 15% to 29% of total cases (**Fig. 4**).[2–5] Although the underlying defect occurs during development, the term "congenital diaphragmatic hernia" is generally preferred for those that appear in the neonatal period, with "Bochdalek hernia" reserved for those that only become apparent in adulthood.[6] Bochdalek hernias are uncommon among adults, with the majority of these hernias found incidentally making the true incidence difficult to surmise.[7] Some reports have suggested a higher prevalence of Bochdalek hernias, perhaps as high as 6%, when data are extrapolated to account for asymptomatic cases.[8]

[a] The Geisel School of Medicine at Dartmouth, 1 Rope Ferry Road, Hanover, NH 03755, USA; [b] Department of Surgery, Section of Thoracic Surgery, Dartmouth-Hitchcock Medical Center, 1 Medical Center Drive, Lebanon, NH 03756, USA; [c] The Dartmouth Institute of Health Policy and Clinical Practice, Williamson Translational Research Building, Level 51 Medical Center Drive, Lebanon, NH 03756, USA
* Corresponding author.
E-mail address: rian.m.hasson@hitchcock.org

Thorac Surg Clin 34 (2024) 155–162
https://doi.org/10.1016/j.thorsurg.2024.01.007

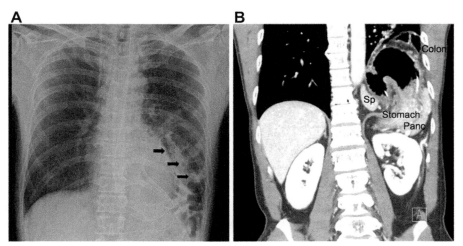

Fig. 1. Case report imaging of a left-sided Bochdalek hernia. Chest X-ray with black arrows demonstrating the presence of bowel above the diaphragm in the left thoracic cavity alongside a nasogastric tube (*A*). Coronal computed tomography image showing abdominal viscera—the stomach, pancreas (panc), spleen (sp) and colon—in the left thoracic cavity (*B*). (*From* M. Akita, N. Yamasaki, T. Miyake, K. Mimura, E. Maeda, T. Nishimura, K. Abe, A. Kozuki, K. Yokoyama, H. Kominami, T. Tanaka, M. Takamatsu and K. Kaneda. Bochdalek Hernia in an Adult: Two Case Reports and a Review of Perioperative Cardiopulmonary Complications. Surgical Case Reports. 2020, 6(1): 72.)

EMBRYOLOGY AND ANATOMY OF THE DIAPHRAGM

Bochdalek hernias are believed to result from a combination of genetic and environmental insults that disrupt normal growth of the pleuroperitoneal fold cells in the developing diaphragm (**Fig. 5**).[9,10] There is active and ongoing research into the genetic pathways and potential genes implicated in the development of diaphragmatic defects, but

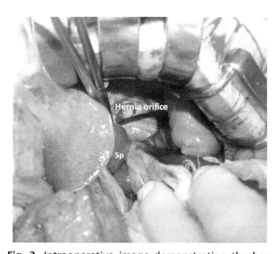

Fig. 2. Intraoperative image demonstrating the hernia orifice without evidence of hernia sac following reduction of abdominal viscera. (*From* M. Akita, N. Yamasaki, T. Miyake, K. Mimura, E. Maeda, T. Nishimura, K. Abe, A. Kozuki, K. Yokoyama, H. Kominami, T. Tanaka, M. Takamatsu and K. Kaneda. Bochdalek Hernia in an Adult: Two Case Reports and a Review of Perioperative Cardiopulmonary Complications. Surgical Case Reports. 2020, 6(1): 72.)

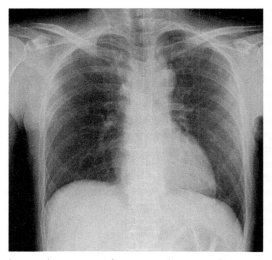

Fig. 3. Chest X-ray after surgical repair of the left-sided Bochdalek hernia showing a fully expanded left lung without radiographic evidence of pleural effusion or pulmonary edema. (*From* M. Akita, N. Yamasaki, T. Miyake, K. Mimura, E. Maeda, T. Nishimura, K. Abe, A. Kozuki, K. Yokoyama, H. Kominami, T. Tanaka, M. Takamatsu and K. Kaneda. Bochdalek Hernia in an Adult: Two Case Reports and a Review of Perioperative Cardiopulmonary Complications. Surgical Case Reports. 2020, 6(1): 72.)

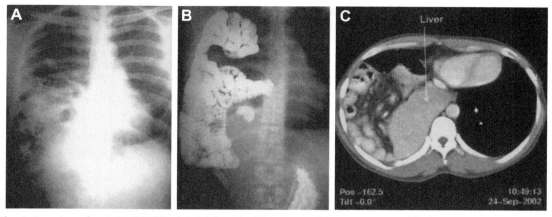

Fig. 4. Imaging of a right-sided Bochdalek hernia. Chest X-ray demonstrating air-filled bowel above the raised right diaphragm (*A*). Upper gastrointestinal barium swallow study revealing the presence of abdominal viscera in the right thoracic cavity (*B*). Contrast-enhanced computed tomography showing abdominal viscera in the posterolateral region of the right thoracic cavity (*C*). (*From* A. Alam and B. N. Chandler. Adult Bochdalek Hernia. Medical journal, Armed Forces India. 2005, 61(3): 284-286.)

that is beyond the scope of this discussion.[11] Embryogenesis of the diaphragm is an incompletely understood process that requires coordinated development of muscular, tendinous, and muscular connective tissues (see Sadia Tasnim and colleagues' article, "Surgical Diaphragm: Anatomy and Physiology," in this issue for a more in depth discussion).[12] A summary of the embryologic process described by Schumpelick and colleagues is as follows.[13]

- The diaphragm is formed from the septum transversum, pleuroperitoneal membranes, mediastinum, and body wall muscles.
- The septum transversum can be seen ventrally at the end of the third week of gestation and is

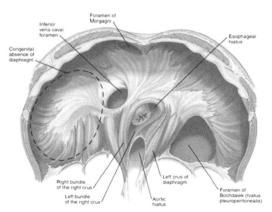

Fig. 5. A schematic diagram of the diaphragm showing the location of congenital and acquired defects. (*From* H. S. W. Haroun, "Congenital Diaphragmatic Hernias: A Review Article," Anatomy Physiology & Biochemistry International Journal, vol. 4, no. 2, p. 555635, 2018.)

a mesodermic mass at the level of the occipital and upper cervical somites (C3).
- As the septum transversum migrates past the third through fifth segments of the neck, it is joined by myogenous stem cells from these somites and myoblasts of the post hepatic plate of mesenchyme.
- Somites 4 and 5 are the origins of nerves that penetrate through the pleuropericardial folds and into the septum transversum during the fifth week of gestation—these will become the phrenic nerves.
- By the eighth week of gestation, the initial diaphragm is at the L1 level, but it does not extend to the dorsal body wall.
  - The communications between the left and right pleural and peritoneal cavities, known as pleuroperitoneal ducts, are closed by the left and right pleuroperitoneal membranes at approximately the end of the eighth week of gestation.
- During weeks 9 to 12 of gestation, the pleural cavities expand to the lateral body wall and penetrate it, forming the costodiaphragmatic recesses and integrating body wall musculature into the diaphragm.
  - The integration of thoracic muscle explains why peripheral parts of the diaphragm are innervated by the lower intercostal nerves.

PATIENT PRESENTATION AND EVALUATION

Gastrointestinal, pulmonary, and cardiac symptomatology are all possible, albeit rare with most patients presenting with non-specific symptoms thereby resulting in the misdiagnosis of many patients presenting with a Bochdalek hernia.[14] There are reports attributing symptoms of Bochdalek hernias to possible diverticulitis, gastric band complications, and even hollow viscus perforation with peritonitis.[15–17] The most common symptoms include pain, chest pressure, dysphagia, dyspepsia, dyspnea, cough, shortness of breath, and even cardiac complaints.[3,4] Late presentation of a congenital weakness in the diaphragm can be precipitated by increased intraabdominal pressure, such as pregnancy, obesity, diving, chronic constipation, and severe coughing.[18] There is even a case attributed to precipitation in a Zumba dance class.[19]

The method of detection and diagnosis of Bochdalek hernias in adults will vary depending on its size. Upon physical examination, larger hernias are more likely to present with decreased breath sounds, increased bowel sounds in the chest, and wheezing.[14,20,21] CT scans are helpful in the accurate detection of Bochdalek hernias and differentiating the hernia from alternate pathology.[22] In his 1985 work, Gale described the following criteria for the CT diagnosis of Bochdalek hernia (**Box 1**).[8]

Additional research has been done looking at posterior traumatic rupture of the diaphragm. Killeen and colleagues found that CT could detect a diaphragm rupture with a sensitivity of 78% and 50% on the left and right sides, respectively.[23,24]

Box 1
Computed tomography criteria for Bochdalek hernia

Detection of a soft-tissue or fatty mass on the thoracic surface of the diaphragm.[a]

Location of the mass in the posteromedial aspect of the hemi diaphragm.

Discontinuity of the muscle of the diaphragm where it meets the mass.

V-shaped diaphragmatic muscle at a point of discontinuity of the diaphragm where it meets the mass.[b]

Congruence and continuity of subdiaphragmatic and supradiaphragmatic densities through the defect in the diaphragm (see **Fig. 1B**).

[a] In 1987, Shin and colleagues add that the round mass should have an attenuation coefficient equal to that of the adipose tissue found on the thoracic surface of the diaphragm (around −130 to −120 Hounsfield units).[23] [b] Shin and colleagues describe the appearance of V-shaped diaphragmatic musculature at the interface of the diaphragm and mass as particularly characteristic of Bochdalek hernias.[23]

Contemporarily, new and improved radiologic techniques, such as 3-dimensional (3D) rendering and maximal intensity projection, have allowed more accurate and complete visualization of the diaphragm and associated defects.[25]

SURGICAL TREATMENT OPTIONS AND COMPLICATIONS

Symptomatic patients with Bochdalek hernias should be recommended to undergo repair. As the true incidence of these hernias is unknown and many are discovered incidentally, there may be a role for watching waiting in some cases, however, this remains poorly defined.[25] Traditionally, repair has been recommended in any hernias to avoid the potential complication of tissue strangulation. Emergent presentations can include gastric perforation and necrosis, small bowel or colon perforation, acute respiratory failure, cardiopulmonary arrest, and hemorrhagic and septic shock.[26–30] Even in an acute setting, with prompt intervention, excellent outcomes can be achieved.[31,32]

There are 5 described surgical approaches to repair a Bochdalek hernia in adults: laparotomy, thoracotomy, laparoscopy, thoracoscopy, and combined.[4] Moro and colleagues emphasize the importance of tailoring the surgical approach to the patient and anatomy of the hernia as no consensus on the optimal approach has been reached, and each has benefits and limitations.[33] A trans-thoracic approach provides an excellent view of the diaphragm, making repair of the hernia orifice and separation of adhesions to the lung, mediastinum, or chest wall easier, but sacrifices visualization of the herniated viscera.[14,33] Contraindications to a thoracic approach include malrotation which should be excluded with imaging prior to proceeding with repair.[34,35]

A transabdominal approach provides excellent access for reduction, evaluation, and management of any complications related to herniated organs, however, provides a more limited view of the thoracic cavity. Inadequate management of the chest can manifest with incomplete pulmonary expansion and postoperative pleural effusions.[33,36] Additionally, a laparoscopic approach can lead to a pneumothorax which can be variably tolerated depending on underlying or comorbid conditions. It is for this reason that Takeyama and colleagues encourage a thoracoscopic approach when possible. To mitigate this risk, a cannula or trocar may be placed in the chest to decompress insufflation and avoid tension physiology.[4] Repair of right-sided Bochdalek hernias is also challenging secondary to the obstruction

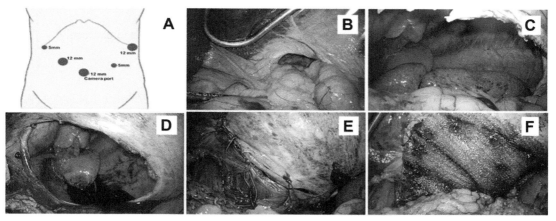

Fig. 6. Use of mesh to repair a diaphragmatic defect. Port sites used for laparoscopic approach (*A*). Left-sided diaphragmatic defect with prolapsed abdominal viscera (*B*). Spleen adhered to the left thoracic cavity (*C*). Exposed defect measuring 10 × 8 cm (*D*). Defect closed with nonabsorbable sutures (*E*). Repair reinforced with mesh (*F*). (*From* Miyasaka T. et al. Laparoscopic repair of a Bochdalek hernia in an elderly patient: a case report with a review from 1999 to 2019 in Japan. (2020) surg case rep. 6:233.)

of the operating field caused by the liver.[37] A rare but notable complication to laparotomy is abdominal compartment syndrome.[38]

A combined thoracoabdominal approach affords the greatest exposure but also carries the greatest associated morbidity.[33]

A minimally invasive approach often confers lower morbidity and a shorter length of stay, but this is not always possible, in particular in emergency setting with strangulated or compromised viscera requiring resection.[4,39] The approach should be selected such that the patient gets the best repair and best access to adequately assess intra-abdominal contents.

The positioning of the patient will depend on both the laterality of the hernia and the approach but is most commonly either a supine position or lateral decubitus helped by reverse Trendelenberg.[4,39,40]

Following the repair of a Bochdalek hernia, recurrence is possible if the strength of the reconstructed diaphragm is insufficient to withstand the perpetual stresses of respiration. To reduce the possibility of failure, defects are often repaired with mesh to achieve a tensionless repair. Many authors favor polytetrafluoroethylene and dual prostheses over polypropylene due to the decreased likelihood of intra-abdominal or thoracic adhesion formation or erosion into abdominal organs (**Fig. 6**).[41–43]

NEW DEVELOPMENTS

In their 2007 article, Meehan and Sandler describe their successful use of the Intuitive Surgical Da Vinci Robot to repair neonatal, congenital Bochdalek hernia.[44] This case remained the only

published report of a robotic repair until a 2015 paper described a successful transabdominal repair of a Bochdalek hernia containing an intrathoracic kidney in an 80-year-old female.[37] More recently, robotic repair of Bochdalek hernias has become increasingly popular through both transthoracic and abdominal approaches with cited benefits of reduced morbidity, enhanced visualization, and improved surgical dexterity and precision.[41,45–48] A robotic approach is likely to become increasingly preferred with more readily available equipment and surgeon experience.[38,47]

MORBIDITY AND MORTALITY

Postoperative complications include pneumonia, pleural effusion, surgical site infection, respiratory failure, and abdominal compartment syndrome in the early post-operative course.[1,3,48] Long-term symptomatic complaints include gastroesophageal reflux, but due to the rarity of the condition there are little long-term patient-reported outcomes available. Mortality ranges from 2.7% to 4.4%; interestingly with rates varying by approach with a laparotomy and thoracotomy portending higher risk.[3,49] This is attributed to the higher rates of open emergent cases.

SUMMARY

Bochdalek hernias in adults are rare in presentation and poorly represented in the literature limiting robust analysis.

As a result of the morbidity and mortality associated with strangulation and urgent repair, the identification of any Bochdalek hernia regardless of symptoms has been recommended to undergo repair. However, major questions remain as to the need for repair in all patients, the optimal timing, approach, and there is a paucity of data on long-term outcomes.

Certainly, advancements in minimally invasive surgical technologies and experience have increased the number of cases being performed by minimally invasive approach and contemporarily laparoscopy and thoracoscopy are preferred when feasible. However, the approach should be selected to afford the greatest visibility and ability to address herniated structures in the safest manner.

CLINICS CARE POINTS

- Bochdalek hernias result from posterolateral defects in diaphragmatic pleuroperitoneal folds.
- These hernias may be clinically silent, found incidentally on CT or MRI.
- In cases presenting with symptoms, they are often non-specific, leading to missed diagnoses or misdiagnoses.
- Computed tomography is the preferred imaging modality.
- Due to the risk of acute mortality or morbidity, it is recommended that even asymptomatic Bochdalek hernias are surgically repaired.
- Surgical approach will depend on anatomy, acuity, and availability.
  - Anatomy: the preferred approach for strangulated hernias with the possibility of resection is through the abdominal cavity, whereas separation of extensive pleural adhesions and easier repair of the hernia orifice is possible with a thoracic approach.
  - Acuity: emergent situations may call for repair with an open approach for efficiency and enhanced access to strangulated contents.
  - Availability: robotic repair is becoming increasingly popular and should be considered under appropriate circumstances and when the required equipment and a robotic-trained surgeon are available.
- Data regarding outcomes are limited, but mortality and morbidity is seemingly higher with open approaches, although this is likely a result of minimally invasive approaches being reserved for healthier patients.

DISCLOSURE

The authors have nothing to disclose.

REFERENCES

1. Akita M, Yamasaki N, Miyake T, et al. Bochdalek Hernia in an Adult: Two Case Reports and a Review of Perioperative Cardiopulmonary Complications. Surgical Case Reports 2020;6(1):72.
2. Alam A, Chandler BN. Adult Bochdalek Hernia. Medical journal, Armed Forces India 2005;61(3):284–6.
3. Katsaros I, Giannopoulos S, Katelani S, et al. Bochdalek Hernias in the Adult Population: a Systematic Review of the Literature. ANZ J Surg 2022;92(9):2037–42.
4. Brown SR, Horton JD, Trivette E, et al. Bochdalek Hernia in the Adult: Demographics, Presentation, and Surgical Management. Hernia : the journal of hernias and abdominal wall surgery 2011;15(1):23–30.
5. Gedik E, Tuncer MC, Onat S, et al. A Review of Morgagni and Bochdalek Hernias in Adults. Folia morphologica 2011;70(1):5–12.
6. Ramos Pachon CM, Broceta A, Dam AM, et al. Symptomatic Right-Sided Bochdalek Hernia in a 91-Year Old Female. Am J Gastroenterol 2022;117(10S):e2301–2.
7. Ivosevic A, Meta-Jevtovic I, Cupurdija V, et al. Bochdalek Hernia in Adults: A Case Report. Vojnosanit Pregl 2018;75(6):628–31.
8. Gale ME. Bochdalek Hernia: Prevalence and CT Characteristics. Radiology 1985;156(2):449–52.
9. Veenma DC, de Klein A, Tibboel D. Developmental and Genetic Aspects of Congenital Diaphragmatic Hernia: Developmental and Genetic Aspects of CDH. Pediatr Pulmonol 2012;47(6):534–45.
10. Haroun HSW. Congenital Diaphragmatic Hernias: A Review Article. Anatomy Physiology & Biochemistry International Journal 2018;4(2):555635.
11. De Leon N, Tse WH, Ameis D, et al. Embryology and Anatomy of Congenital Diaphragmatic Hernia. Semin Pediatr Surg 2022;31(6):151229.
12. Merrell AJ, Ellis BJ, Fox ZD, et al. Muscle Connective Tissue Controls Development of the Diaphragm and Is a Source of Congenital Diaphragmatic Hernias. Nat Genet 2015;47(5):496–504.
13. Schumpelick V, Steinau G, Schluper I, et al. Surgical Embryology and Anatomy of the Diaphragm with Surgical Applications. Surg Clin 2000;80(1):213–39.
14. Zhou Y, Du H, Che G. Giant Congenital Diaphragmatic Hernia in an Adult. J Cardiothorac Surg 2014;9(2):31.
15. Tan CQY, Chan DL, Chu F, et al. Rare Presentation of a Bochdalek Hernia in Adulthood with Incarcerated Splenic Flexure of the Colon Mimicking Diverticulitis:

a Report and Review. ANZ J Surg 2019;89(11): 1518–20.

16. Rapti N, Kanakis M, Misthos P, et al. An Unusual Presentation of Bochdalek Hernia after Laparoscopic Surgery. Hellenic journal of surgery 2016;88(3): 208–10.

17. Kumar A, Maheshwari V, Ramakrishnan T, et al. Caecal Perforation with Faecal Peritonitis - Unusual Presentation of Bochdalek Hernia in an Adult: A Case Report and Review of Literature. World J Emerg Surg 2009;4(1):16.

18. Choi J-Y, Yang S-S, Lee J-H, et al. Maternal Bochdalek Hernia During Pregnancy: A Systematic Review of Case Reports. Diagnostics 2021;11(7):1261.

19. Rehman A, Maliyakkal AM, Naushad VA, et al. A Lady with Severe Abdominal Pain Following a Zumba Dance Session: A Rare Presentation of Bochdalek Hernia. Curēus (Palo Alto, CA) 2018; 10(4):e2427.

20. Venkatesh SP, Ravi MJ, Thrishuli PB, et al. Asymptomatic Presentation of Bochdalek's Hernia in an Adult. Indian journal of surgery 2011;73(5):382–3.

21. Mohammed S, El-Basheir H. Obstructed Bochdalek Hernia in an Adult. Oxford Medical Case Reports 2022;2022(12):omac138.

22. Kikuchi S, Nishizaki M, Kuroda S, et al. A Case of Right-Sided Bochdalek Hernia Incidentally Diagnosed in a Gastric Cancer Patient. BMC Surg 2016;16(1):34.

23. Shin MS, Mulligan SA, Baxley WA, et al. Bochdalek Hernia of Diaphragm in the Adult. Diagnosis by Computed Tomography. Chest 1987;92(6): 1098–101.

24. Killeen KL, Mirvis SE, Shanmuganathan K. Helical CT of Diaphragmatic Rupture Caused by Blunt Trauma. American journal of roentgenology (1976) 1999;173(6):1611–6.

25. Mullins ME, Saini S. Imaging of Incidental Bochdalek Hernia. Seminars in ultrasound, CT, and MRI 2005; 26(1):28–36.

26. Chui PP, Tan CT. Sudden death due to incarcerated Bochdalek hernia in an adult. Ann Acad Med Singapore 1993;22(1):57–60.

27. Kanazawa A, Yoshioka Y, Inoi O, et al. Acute Respiratory Failure Caused by an Incarcerated Right-Sided Adult Bochdalek Hernia: Report of a Case. Surgery today (Tokyo, Japan) 2002;32(9):812–5.

28. Machado Contreras LA, Retamoso Díaz SP, Valencia G, et al. Sudden Onset Dyspnea Caused by Bochdalek Diaphragmatic Hernia in an Adult: a Case Report. J Med Case Rep 2021;15(1):424.

29. Živković V, Cvetković D, Atanasijević T, et al. Ectopic Right Thoracic Kidney Associated with Bochdalek Hernia as the Cause of Diagnostic Confusion. Forensic Sci Med Pathol 2021;17(3):456–60.

30. Eslamian M, Goharian M, Ghasempour Dabaghi G, et al. Obstructed Descending Colon Mass Presented With Bochdalek Hernia: A Case Report. Clin Med Insights Case Rep 2023;16.

31. Losanoff JE, Sauter ER. Congenital Posterolateral Diaphragmatic Hernia in an Adult. Hernia : the journal of hernias and abdominal wall surgery 2004;8(1): 83–5.

32. Halle-Smith JM, Pande R, Griffiths EA. Urgent Surgical Repair of Symptomatic Bochdalek Hernia Containing an Intrathoracic Kidney. Ann R Coll Surg Engl 2021;103(1):E10–2.

33. Moro K, Kawahara M, Muneoka Y, et al. Right-Sided Bochdalek Hernia in an Elderly Adult: a Case Report with a Review of Surgical Management. Surgical Case Reports 2017;3(1):109.

34. Enomoto N, Yamada K, Kato D, et al. Right-Sided Bochdalek Hernia in an Adult with Hepatic Malformation and Intestinal Malrotation. Surgical Case Reports 2021;7(1):169.

35. Silen ML, Canvasser DA, Kurkchubasche AG, et al. Video-Assisted Thoracic Surgical Repair of a Foramen of Bochdalek Hernia. Ann Thorac Surg 1995; 60(2):448–50.

36. Suzuki T, Okamoto T, Hanyu K, et al. Repair of Bochdalek Hernia in an Adult Complicated by Abdominal Compartment Syndrome, Gastropleural Fistula and Pleural Empyema: Report of a Case. International Journal of Surgery Case Reports 2014;5(2):82–5.

37. Chen B, Finnerty BM, Schamberg NJ, et al. Transabdominal Robotic Repair of a Congenital Right Diaphragmatic Hernia Containing an Intrathoracic Kidney: a Case Report. Journal of Robotic Surgery 2015;9(4):357–60.

38. Dalencourt G, Katlic MR. Abdominal compartment syndrome after late repair of bochdalek hernia. Ann Thorac Surg 2006;82(2):721–2.

39. Lau N-S, Crawford M, Sandroussi C. Surgical Management of Symptomatic Right-sided Bochdalek Hernias in Adults: When Is a Minimally Invasive Approach Appropriate? ANZ J Surg 2020;90(6): 1075–9.

40. Shen Y-G, Jiao N-N, Xiong W, et al. Video-Assisted Thoracoscopic Surgery for Adult Bochdalek Hernia: a Case Report. J Cardiothorac Surg 2016;11(1):165.

41. Kozadinos A, Chrysikos D, Davakis S, et al. Bochdalek Hernia with Intrathoracic Spleen Treated by Robotic-Assisted Mesh Repair Utilizing Indocyanine Green Contrast Media Intraoperatively. A Case Report. J Surg Case Rep 2021;2021(8).

42. Takeyama K, Nakahara Y, Ando S, et al. Anesthetic Management for Repair of Adult Bochdalek Hernia by Laparoscopic Surgery. J Anesth 2005;19(1): 78–80.

43. Yagmur Y, Yiğit E, Babur M, et al. Bochdalek Hernia: A Rare Case Report of Adult Age. Annals of Medicine and Surgery 2016;5:72–5.

44. Meehan JJ, Sandler A. Robotic Repair of a Bochdalek Congenital Diaphragmatic Hernia in a Small

Neonate: Robotic Advantages and Limitations. J Pediatr Surg 2007;42(10):1757–60.

45. Jambhekar A, Robinson S, Housman B, et al. Robotic Repair of a Right-Sided Bochdalek Hernia: a Case Report and Literature Review. Journal of Robotic Surgery 2018;12(2):351–5.

46. Doamba RN, Cherqui D, Bazongo M, et al. Bochdalek hernia with intrathoracic liver herniation in an adult patient treated with robotic surgery: a case report. The Pan African Medical Journal 2021;39.

47. Sidhu KK, Van Kessel CS, Cao C, et al. The Combination of Chilaiditi Syndrome and Bochdalek Hernia in an Adult: Successful Management with a Robot Assisted Approach. ANZ J Surg 2023;93(4):1035–7.

48. Machado NO. Laparoscopic Repair of Bochdalek Diaphragmatic Hernia in Adults. N Am J Med Sci 2016;8(2):65–74.

49. Miyasaka T, Matsutani T, Nomura T, et al. Laparoscopic repair of a Bochdalek hernia in an elderly patient: a case report with a review from 1999 to 2019 in Japan. Surg Case Rep 2020;6:233.

Management of Paraesophageal Hernias

Ryan J. Randle, MD[a,b,1], Douglas Z. Liou, MD[b], Natalie S. Lui, MD[b,*]

KEYWORDS

- Paraesophageal hernia • Fundoplication • Hiatal hernia • Gastroesophageal reflux disease
- Dysphagia

KEY POINTS

- All patients with symptomatic paraesophageal hernias should undergo elective operation.
- Achieving 3 cm of esophageal length and performance of a fundoplication are crucial to repair.
- Symptoms rather than radiographic findings should serve as the mainstay for assessing recurrence.

INTRODUCTION

Hiatal hernias represent a migration of the gastroesophageal junction (GEJ) and/or portions of the abdominal visceral contents into the mediastinum. These hernias are classified into four types (I–IV) to reflect the altered anatomic relationship between the esophageal hiatus, GEJ, and stomach. Type I hernias, also termed "sliding," reflect migration of the GEJ junction above the esophageal hiatus and into the mediastinum. This is the most common type and is often present in patients suffering from gastroesophageal reflux disease (GERD). Type II hiatal hernias refer to those where the gastric fundus protrudes into the mediastinum, but the GEJ remains in its usual intra-abdominal position. Type III hernias are a combination of types I and II, herniation of both the stomach and GEJ. Type IV hernias occur when the stomach along with an additional intra-abdominal organ such as the colon, liver, or spleen is also displaced into the chest. Types II–IV are separately referred to as paraesophageal hernias (PEHs) and share the defining feature of herniated stomach in the mediastinum. In addition, some surgeons describe hernias that contain greater than 50% of the body of the stomach as "giant," although this sizing definition is not consistent throughout the literature.

PRESENTATION
Symptomatic

Symptoms associated with PEH can be wide ranging.[1] Many patients present with heartburn or regurgitation that may otherwise be attributed to typical GERD symptoms.[2,3] Atypical symptoms of GERD such as respiratory complaints (eg, cough, dyspnea, wheezing) and dysphagia are also present among many patients.[4] As these hernias enlarge, the onset of increased mass effect on the mediastinum and mechanical obstruction produces chest pain, postprandial bloating and can progress to complete gastric outlet obstruction in rare cases.

Asymptomatic

It is recognized that not everyone with a PEH will be symptomatic, as many are identified on noninvasive imaging for other reasons. Although the exact number of asymptomatic PEHs is not known, some investigators believe that asymptomatic patients make up as many as half of all PEHs.[5] Alternatively, because the symptoms described above are nonspecific and occasionally mild, it is debated whether patients may simply fail to recognize these symptoms rather than truly have absent symptoms.

[a] Department of Surgery, Oregon Health and Science University, 3181 Southwest Sam Jackson Park Road, Mail Code L223, Portland, OR, USA; [b] Division of Thoracic Surgery, Department of Cardiothoracic Surgery, Stanford School of Medicine, 300 Pasteur Drive, Falk Building, Stanford, CA 94305, USA
[1] Present address: 3181 Southwest Sam Jackson Park Road Mail Code: L223, Portland, OR 97239.
* Corresponding author. 300 Pasteur Drive, Falk Building, Stanford, CA 94305.
E-mail address: natalielui@stanford.edu
Twitter: @radonrandle (R.J.R.); @DouglasLiou (D.Z.L.); @natalielui22 (N.S.L.)

Thorac Surg Clin 34 (2024) 163–170
https://doi.org/10.1016/j.thorsurg.2024.01.005
1547-4127/24/© 2024 Elsevier Inc. All rights reserved.

PREOPERATIVE WORKUP
Indications

Symptoms
Most recent guidelines recommend any patient presenting with symptoms attributable to a PEH undergo elective operative repair.[6] Indeed, several studies have identified that elective repair of PEHs reliably improves symptoms in most patients with perioperative mortality rates less than 1%.[1,4,7,8] In surgically fit patients, an elective repair is highly recommended as there is a demonstrable increase in morbidity and mortality, length of stay, and hospital cost associated with emergent PEH repair.[9-11]

Asymptomatic
Given worse outcomes in the setting of emergent repair and the tendency for these hernias to enlarge, some have advocated for the repair of all PEHs regardless of the presence of symptoms. However, this approach remains controversial given that the true number of patients with asymptomatic hernias remains unknown—limiting surgeon ability to describe the natural history of asymptomatic hernias and attendant outcomes. Further, studies modeling a watchful-waiting approach using data on operative mortality, recurrence rates, need for reoperation, and progression to symptomatic hernia have reported that watchful waiting is a superior initial approach to patients with asymptomatic PEHs.[12,13] Ultimately, patient fitness, surgical risks, and willingness to avoid a potential emergent or urgent operation should guide the choice to pursue elective repair of asymptomatic PEHs.

Preoperative Studies

Contrast esophagram
Identifying the anatomic relationship between the herniated stomach and esophageal hiatus is important to establish before operative repair. Contrast esophagram with dilute barium can be performed to establish the diagnosis for this purpose. In addition, assessment of esophageal peristalsis and contrast transit time are useful in the detection of underlying motility disorders. Cross-sectional imaging such as computed tomography (CT) is useful in determining the presence of volvulus or assisting with operative planning (eg, identifying organs involved in a suspected Type IV hernia). Although the presence of a PEH can be suggested on studies such as upright chest x-ray, plain radiograph does not provide sufficient detail for operative planning and definitive diagnosis.

Upper endoscopy
We perform upper endoscopy to evaluate the esophageal and gastric mucosa, presence of linear gastric erosions or ulcers that can occur with hiatal hernias (Cameron lesions), as well as complications associated with chronic GERD such as esophagitis or stricture. After nasogastric decompression, endoscopy is critical in the setting of acute gastric outlet obstruction to identify the presence of gastric necrosis that would warrant resection rather than repair.

Manometry
High-resolution esophageal manometry can be beneficial in the preoperative evaluation of esophageal dysmotility. Repair of the hernia defect followed by Nissen fundoplication in the setting of esophageal dysmotility may substantially contribute to postoperative dysphagia.[14] As a result, manometric confirmation of a significant underlying dysmotility disorder or preoperative dysphagia should discourage the performance of a full fundoplication at the time of repair. In the case of large PEHs, however, correct placement and therefore interpretability of these studies are challenging due to the altered anatomy.[15]

Ambulatory pH
Although a mainstay in the workup for GERD, ambulatory pH monitoring is not essential in patients with symptomatic PEH. However, in patients with vague symptoms that are not attributable to reflux, pH monitoring remains a standard modality for establishing the diagnosis of GERD.

LAPAROSCOPIC SURGICAL APPROACH
Preoperative Endoscopy

We recommend preoperative and intraoperative endoscopy before procedure to aid in assessment of the location of the gastroesophageal junction, undiagnosed lesions (eg, Barrett's esophagus, stricture, or Cameron ulcer), and viability of the gastric mucosa. This can be performed after anesthesia induction and before abdominal preparation. Attention should also be paid to minimizing insufflation and evaluating any potential obstruction to the passage of a bougie during the operation.

Positioning

Patient positioning for this procedure is supine with both arms out, though the left arm can be tucked if desired. A footboard is placed at the feet to accommodate steep reverse-Trendelenburg during the visualization of the hiatus. The operating surgeon is on the patient's right, whereas the assistant stands on the left. Lithotomy position is a variation on positioning allowing the surgeon to stand between the patient's legs with assistant to the left.

Port Placement and Entry

We often perform closed abdominal entry and insufflation using the Veress technique in the left upper quadrant. Following insufflation, the first trocar is a 5-mm camera port roughly two finger-breadths above and to the anatomic left of the umbilicus (**Fig. 1**).

Liver Retraction

A subxiphoid incision is made to insert a liver retractor and elevate the left lateral segment away from the stomach to aid in visualizing the esophageal hiatus (**Fig. 2**). Following this, the patient is gradually placed in steep reverse-Trendelenburg. The remaining ports are a 10 or 12 mm working port opposite the camera port, along with two 5 mm trocars on the right and left lateral aspects of the abdomen.

Hernia Sac Reduction

Contents of the hernia sac may reduce with steep reverse-Trendelenburg. Otherwise, atraumatic graspers are used to grasp the esophageal fat pad to gently reduce the contents of the hernia back into the abdominal cavity. To avoid injury to the underlying vagus nerve, the fat pad or phrenoesophageal membrane is often safely grasped at the 12 o'clock position.

Identification and Dissection of the Right Crus

After successful reduction of hernia contents, we begin the dissection by identification and dissection of the right crus away from the esophagus. We begin with division of the gastrohepatic ligament near the crus—taking care to evaluate for the presence of a replaced left hepatic artery or vagal branches before any division (**Fig. 3**). While maintaining gentle traction on the fat pad or stomach, the peritoneum medial to the right crus is incised and bluntly separated from the esophagus and endothoracic fascia to gain entry into the mediastinum and begin dissection of the attached hernia sac (**Fig. 4**A). Entry into the mediastinum

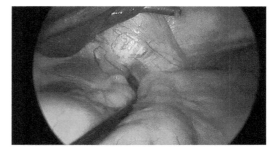

Fig. 2. View of the diaphragmatic hiatus and associated paraesophageal hernia.

should reveal thin areolar tissue that is easily divided with ultrasonic shears or bipolar energy with the goal of complete dissection of the sac from the esophagus and mediastinum (**Fig. 4**B). During this dissection, it is important to look for the pleural reflection to avoid injury to the pleura and subsequent capnothorax. Physiologically, this can result in an initial rise in end-tidal CO_2 which can suddenly transition to hemodynamic instability with the onset of tension physiology. The presence of a large capnothorax is easily identified by enlarging pleura within the mediastinum or bulging of the ipsilateral hemidiaphragm. If physiologic derangement or obstruction of the mediastinum is present, a larger opening can be made into the pleural to equalize pressures and allow for extrusion of CO_2, alternative considerations including introducing a small catheter into the tear to decompress the capnothorax or a pigtail catheter can be externally placed into the chest to evacuate the accumulated CO_2.

Posterior Dissection

Dissection should free the esophagus from posterior adhesions and be carried clockwise to completely mobilize the hernia sac. Satisfactory posterior dissection should allow visualization into the mediastinum and at least partial visualization of the left crus body. Care should be taken to limit dissection directly over the body of the crural

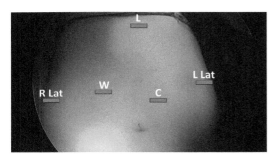

Fig. 1. Laparoscopic incisions for paraesophageal hernia repair. C, camera trocar; L, liver retractor; L Lat, left lateral trocar; R Lat, right lateral trocar; W, working trocar.

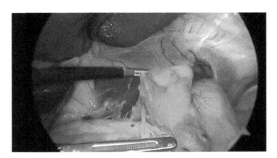

Fig. 3. Division of the gastrohepatic ligament.

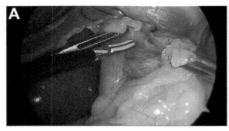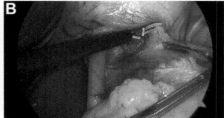

Fig. 4. (*A, B*) Dissection of the hernia sac and entry into the mediastinum.

pillars to avoid damage that would jeopardize the integrity of the repair.

Division of Short Gastric Vessels, Dissection of Left Crus, and Mediastinal Dissection

Following the right crural dissection, the short gastric vessels are divided and the anteromedial aspect of the left crus is similarly dissected away from the esophagus (**Fig. 5**). To provide more forceful atraumatic retraction, a Penrose drain can then be passed through the retroesophageal window and looped around the GEJ. With the esophagus completely mobilized from the bilateral crura and the hiatus exposed, high-mediastinal dissection of the esophagus is performed. Deliberate dissection is taken to ensure preservation of the anterior and posterior branches of the vagus, as well as hemostasis when dividing small vessel branches which may emanate from the aorta (**Fig. 6**). The dissection can be taken to the level of the inferior pulmonary veins for maximal intra-abdominal esophageal length.

Assessment of Esophageal Length

Once the mediastinal dissection is complete, the surgeon must make an assessment of esophageal length and position of the GEJ. A 3 cm of intra-abdominal length should be achieved to avoid tension and maintain the GEJ within the abdomen (**Fig. 7**). Especially in the reoperative setting, external landmarks may prove challenging to identify the GEJ. Transillumination and palpation during intraoperative endoscopy can be helpful to visually confirm the transition from esophagus to stomach in this setting.

If 3 cm of length cannot be achieved despite thorough dissection, we perform a Collis-type gastroplasty as follows to lengthen the esophagus.

- A 54-Fr bougie is placed into the esophagus and advanced into the gastric antrum under direct laparoscopic visualization
- The greater curve of the stomach is retracted toward the patient's feet and to the left so the bougie lays along the lesser curve. An endoscopic stapler (45 or 60 mm) is fired across the fundus perpendicular to the bougie.
- Successive fires are made parallel to the bougie and toward the GEJ to complete the wedge resection of the stomach.

Crural Closure

With sufficient intra-abdominal esophageal length, the crura are subsequently reapproximated. We prefer a simple interrupted technique with braided, 0-suture proceeding from the most posterior aspect of the crura anteriorly (**Fig. 8**). The crura should be closed around the distal esophagus until an instrument can barely be passed into the mediastinum with a bougie inside the esophagus.

Reapproximating the crura can prove challenging in the case of large chronic hernias and redo repairs. One option is using mesh to buttress

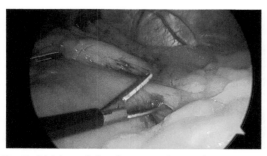

Fig. 5. Division of the short gastric vessels.

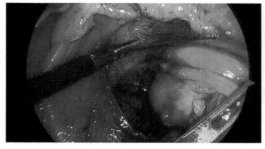

Fig. 6. High-mediastinal dissection.

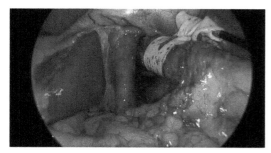

Fig. 7. Assessment of intra-abdominal esophageal length.

or bridge the crura. An absorbable biologic mesh is preferred to avoid mesh erosion at the GEJ. Another option is using relaxing diaphragm incisions that are then repaired with a patch (eg, Gore-Tex).[16] A right relaxing incision must allow enough space from the inferior vena cava to safely close the defect, whereas a left relaxing incision must avoid the phrenic nerve. Prior surgery or expected adhesions in one hemithorax may also guide selected laterality.

Fundoplication

The choice to perform a partial fundoplication (eg, Dor or Toupet) versus a Nissen is dictated by the presence of esophageal dysmotility, severe dysphagia, or other patient factors.

A traditional wrap or Nissen is a 360° wrap. After mobilization of the esophagus and stomach and closure of the hiatus, the fundus of the stomach is passed posteriorly around the esophagus from left to right. A second most distal site along the greater curve is grasped and shoeshine maneuver performed — the fundoplication slid back and forth behind the esophagus assuring the stomach to be in good position without twisting or redundancy. With a bougie in place, three sutures are placed taking full-thickness bites through each side of the fundoplication and incorporating a partial thickness bite of the esophagus to create a 2-cm wrap sitting just above the GEJ. On completion of the wrap, the bougie should be withdrawn and wrap assessed to

assure appropriate position and no excess tension that could precipitate dysphagia.

In the presence of features which predispose patients to severe postoperative dysphagia, a Toupet fundoplication may be performed over a large bougie. With the bougie in place, the cephalad aspect of the fundus is grasped and wrapped 270° around the posterior of the esophagus. The fundus is positioned to partially cover the left and right anterior edges of the esophagus. On each side, we use braided 0-suture to place interrupted stitches from the anterior edge of the fundus to the esophagus along its 3 cm length. The bougie is removed, and the final results should demonstrate a 270° wrap of the fundus that leaves the anterior aspect of the esophagus exposed (**Fig. 9**). Once the Toupet is fashioned, the procedure is concluded with an intraoperative endoscopy that should identify 270° of concentric gastric mucosa around the posterior aspect of the GEJ.

A final approach is the Dor fundoplication or partial anterior wrap. The fundus of the stomach is folded from left to right over the anterior esophagus and secured to both the esophagus and diaphragmatic hiatus generally beginning on the left crus and proceeding in a counter-clockwise direction with interrupted braided sutures. Keys to success include the recreation of the angle of His with the first or second stitch incorporating the fundus and left crus of the diaphragm and avoiding twisting of the distal esophagus, GEJ, or cardia. A Dor like the Nissen or Toupet may be performed over a Bougie or an endoscope.

TRANSTHORACIC APPROACH

Laparoscopic and robotic approaches to abdominal repair of PEHs are the dominant approach in modern surgery. However, transthoracic approaches are still used in select circumstances. Transthoracic repair is mostly performed through a thoracotomy, which causes the surgeon to forfeit the benefits of minimally invasive surgery. However, the substantial visualization of the intrathoracic esophagus and avoidance of potentially tenacious

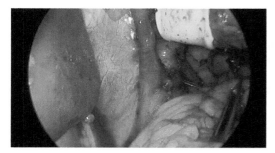

Fig. 8. Posterior closure of the crura.

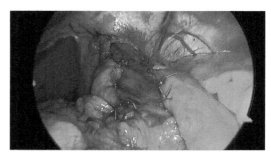

Fig. 9. Completed Toupet fundoplication.

adhesions from previous abdominal operations makes this a very attractive approach in patients undergoing revisional surgery from recurrent esophageal hernias.[17]

POSTOPERATIVE CARE
Hospital Care and Follow-Up

Postoperatively, patients are typically extubated and transferred to the ward or intensive care unit if patient's condition and comorbidities dictate. Patients are maintained nil per os (NPO) with maintenance fluids on the day of operation. On the first postoperative day, we routinely perform a swallow esophagram. This provides a baseline assessment of contrast transit through the GEJ in the evaluation of any postoperative dysphagia, as well as possible early recurrence. Although uncommon even among repairs of large hernias, esophagrams also identify the presence of possible leak. If no leak or recurrence is identified, patients should be transitioned to a small volume, clear liquid diet and intravenous fluids should be discontinued. In our practice, patients that receive a Collis-type gastroplasty remain NPO until postoperative day 2, at which time an unremarkable esophagram should also prompt transition to a clear liquid diet. Following acceptable pain control and ability to tolerate clear liquids for 24 hours, patients may be discharged home on a full liquid diet with clinic follow-up within 10 to 14 days.

Nausea is common in the early postoperative period and should be treated intensively with intravenous antiemetic medication to prevent retching and subsequent damage to the hernia repair. Multimodal pain control and treatment of gas bloat are mainstays to increase patient comfort. Similarly, opioid analgesia is used sparingly to limit potential for opioid-induced constipation and abdominal discomfort.

Postoperative Complications

Some relevant postoperative complications include bleeding, early recurrence, and esophageal obstruction. Esophageal perforation should be considered if patients have any associated symptoms or signs, especially after reoperative cases in which the anatomy around the GEJ can be unclear. Overall, the complication rates of entities, such as deep venous thrombosis, pneumonia, bleeding, and need for re-operative intervention, are low.[8,18]

OUTCOMES
Recurrences and Symptomatic Improvement

At 1 year, contrast esophagram is used to assess for radiographic recurrence of PEH. Studies often use a threshold of greater than 2 cm of gastric mucosa above the diaphragm to diagnose recurrence.[7,19] However, even with the presence of a small recurrence, many patients remain asymptomatic. Several studies demonstrate that patients with radiographic recurrence demonstrate similar quality of life outcomes compared with those with no radiographic recurrence after follow-up ranging from 1 to 10 years.[19–21] Recurrence rates have been documented as high as 27% on contrast esophagram within the first year despite a statistically significant improvement in patient-reported quality of life after surgery.[19] In contrast to radiographic recurrence, symptomatic recurrence requiring reoperation is less common. In a large retrospective study by Le Page and colleagues, 4.8% (22/455) of patients required revision surgery with a median follow-up of 32 months.[20] These data show that repair of PEHs offers patients substantial symptomatic improvement, and patient-reported symptoms should remain the principal component of managing a potential hernia recurrence.

Reflux, Esophagitis, and Dysphagia

Despite generally excellent symptomatic results from PEH repair, issues with reflux and dysphagia may persist. Indeed, dysphagia is a common presenting symptom of patients with PEH, and its presence predicts postoperative dysphagia among patients undergoing repair and fundoplication.[14] Although Le Page and colleagues' study did not demonstrate improvement in dysphagia at short- or long-term follow-up, this finding seems to be inconsistent with other literature. More likely, dysphagia is predominantly related to features of the operative repair such as postsurgical swelling or altered anatomy (eg, reduction of herniated tissue or fundoplication). Bernard and colleagues retrospectively reviewed 85 patients that underwent hiatal repair and fundoplication and discovered that 15% of patients had new-onset dysphagia, though the cohort overall demonstrated a statistically significant decrease in dysphagia.[21] Similarly, Li and colleagues provide evidence that postoperative dysphagia—especially as it relates to performance of fundoplication—seems to gradually resolve in patients over the course of several months.[22]

Despite the apparent increase in dysphagia that is reported with performance of fundoplication, we believe it is an important tool in attempting to restore the stomach's anti-reflux mechanism. The study by Li and colleagues importantly demonstrates that patients who underwent hiatal hernia repair (one-third of which were types II–IV) with fundoplication had decreased symptomatic heartburn, esophagitis, and DeMeester scores compared with patients who did not receive fundoplication. Literature demonstrating the presence of postoperative esophagitis and even Barrett's esophagus among these patients highlights the need for long-term studies to better inform recommendations on surveillance.[20,22] Given the current literature, fundoplication seems to provide benefits not realized with crural repair alone—albeit with higher rates of short-term dysphagia.

CONTROVERSIES
Use of Collis

The practice of performing a Collis gastroplasty to increase intra-abdominal esophageal length has been debated among surgeons, some even questioning the existence of a truly shortened esophagus in the context of a hiatal hernia repair.[23] In addition to concerns about increased dysphagia and acid production, some studies have also identified an increase in the rate of postoperative leaks among patients receiving Collis gastroplasty.[7,24] Despite these concerns, the literature supports the use of a Collis-type technique when 3 cm of tension-free, intra-abdominal esophageal length cannot be obtained. Studies by Nason and colleagues and Weltz and colleagues, as well as others demonstrate that patients report comparable quality of life whether or not they receive a Collis gastroplasty after fundoplication during hiatal and PEH repair.[24–26] A Collis should not supplant the need for adequate dissection and mediastinal mobilization of the esophagus; however, if persisting finding of insufficient intra-abdominal esophageal length is identified, the patient should be considered for Collis gastroplasty.

Use of Mesh

The use of mesh is controversial in the repair of PEHs. Our experience dictates that the routine use of mesh is not required to buttress hiatal repair. Further, Oelschlager and colleagues report on long-term results from a randomized controlled trial of patients assigned to hiatal repair with or without biologic mesh for PEH.[27] With 72 of 108 patients available for 5-year follow-up, they report that there was no statistically significant difference in the rates of radiographic recurrence or quality of life. Similar results were obtained from a retrospective study performed by Dallemagne and colleagues with a median follow-up of more than 8 years, demonstrating that mesh did not seem to improve quality of life or recurrence rates.[21] As

a result, we advocate for primary closure without mesh reinforcement in the repair of routine PEHs.

CLINICS CARE POINTS

- Paraesophageal hernia repair is indicated for all symptomatic patients and can be considered for asymptomatic patients with low surgical risk to prevent the need for emergent repair.
- Important steps of paraesophageal hernia repair include dissection of the entire hernia sac and achieving 3 cm esophagus in the abdomen.
- Choosing a partial versus full fundoplication largely depends on manometry and preoperative dysphagia.

DISCLOSURE

The authors have no financial interests or relationships to disclose.

REFERENCES

1. Carrott PW, Hong J, Kuppusamy M, et al. Clinical ramifications of giant paraesophageal hernias are underappreciated: making the case for routine surgical repair. Ann Thorac Surg 2012;94(2):421–6 [discussion 426-428].
2. Mattar SG, Bowers SP, Galloway KD, et al. Long-term outcome of laparoscopic repair of paraesophageal hernia. Surg Endosc 2002;16(5):745–9.
3. Lazar DJ, Birkett DH, Brams DM, et al. Long-Term Patient-Reported Outcomes of Paraesophageal Hernia Repair. Jsls 2017;21(4).
4. Low DE, Simchuk EJ. Effect of paraesophageal hernia repair on pulmonary function. Ann Thorac Surg 2002;74(2):333–7 [discussion 337].
5. Schieman C, Grondin SC. Paraesophageal hernia: clinical presentation, evaluation, and management controversies. Thorac Surg Clin 2009;19(4):473–84.
6. Kohn GP, Price RR, DeMeester SR, et al. Guidelines for the management of hiatal hernia. Surg Endosc 2013;27(12):4409–28.
7. Luketich JD, Nason KS, Christie NA, et al. Outcomes after a decade of laparoscopic giant paraesophageal hernia repair. J Thorac Cardiovasc Surg 2010;139(2):395–404, 404.e391.
8. Mungo B, Molena D, Stem M, et al. Thirty-day outcomes of paraesophageal hernia repair using the NSQIP database: should laparoscopy be the standard of care? J Am Coll Surg 2014;219(2):229–36.

9. Polomsky M, Hu R, Sepesi B, et al. A population-based analysis of emergent vs. elective hospital admissions for an intrathoracic stomach. Surg Endosc 2010;24(6):1250–5.

10. Kaplan JA, Schecter S, Lin MY, et al. Morbidity and Mortality Associated With Elective or Emergency Paraesophageal Hernia Repair. JAMA Surg 2015; 150(11):1094–6.

11. Wong LY, Parsons N, David EA, et al. The impact of age and need for emergent surgery in paraesophageal hernia repair outcomes. Ann Thorac Surg 2023.

12. Stylopoulos N, Gazelle GS, Rattner DW. Paraesophageal hernias: operation or observation? Ann Surg 2002;236(4):492–500 [discussion 500-491].

13. Jung JJ, Naimark DM, Behman R, et al. Approach to asymptomatic paraesophageal hernia: watchful waiting or elective laparoscopic hernia repair? Surg Endosc 2018;32(2):864–71.

14. Kapadia S, Osler T, Lee A, et al. The role of preoperative high resolution manometry in predicting dysphagia after laparoscopic Nissen fundoplication. Surg Endosc 2018;32(5):2365–72.

15. Roman S, Kahrilas PJ, Kia L, et al. Effects of large hiatal hernias on esophageal peristalsis. Arch Surg 2012;147(4):352–7.

16. Greene CL, DeMeester SR, Zehetner J, et al. Diaphragmatic relaxing incisions during laparoscopic paraesophageal hernia repair. Surg Endosc 2013; 27(12):4532–8.

17. Reinersman JM, Deb SJ. Transthoracic Paraesophageal Hernia Repair. Thorac Surg Clin 2019;29(4): 437–46.

18. Andujar JJ, Papasavas PK, Birdas T, et al. Laparoscopic repair of large paraesophageal hernia is associated with a low incidence of recurrence and reoperation. Surg Endosc 2004;18(3):444–7.

19. Lidor AO, Steele KE, Stem M, et al. Long-term quality of life and risk factors for recurrence after laparoscopic repair of paraesophageal hernia. JAMA Surg 2015;150(5):424–31.

20. Le Page PA, Furtado R, Hayward M, et al. Durability of giant hiatus hernia repair in 455 patients over 20 years. Ann R Coll Surg Engl 2015;97(3):188–93.

21. Dallemagne B, Kohnen L, Perretta S, et al. Laparoscopic repair of paraesophageal hernia. Long-term follow-up reveals good clinical outcome despite high radiological recurrence rate. Ann Surg 2011; 253(2):291–6.

22. Li ZT, Ji F, Han XW, et al. Role of fundoplication in treatment of patients with symptoms of hiatal hernia. Sci Rep 2019;9(1):12544.

23. Madan AK, Frantzides CT, Patsavas KL. The myth of the short esophagus. Surg Endosc 2004;18(1): 31–4.

24. Nason KS, Luketich JD, Awais O, et al. Quality of life after Collis gastroplasty for short esophagus in patients with paraesophageal hernia. Ann Thorac Surg 2011;92(5):1854–60 [discussion 1860-1851].

25. Weltz AS, Zahiri HR, Sibia US, et al. Patients are well served by Collis gastroplasty when indicated. Surgery 2017;162(3):568–76.

26. Lu R, Addo A, Broda A, et al. Update on the Durability and Performance of Collis Gastroplasty For Chronic GERD and Hiatal Hernia Repair At 4-Year Post-Intervention. J Gastrointest Surg 2020;24(2): 253–61.

27. Oelschlager BK, Pellegrini CA, Hunter JG, et al. Biologic prosthesis to prevent recurrence after laparoscopic paraesophageal hernia repair: long-term follow-up from a multicenter, prospective, randomized trial. J Am Coll Surg 2011; 213(4):461–8.

Management of Traumatic Diaphragmatic Injuries

Devin Gillaspie, MD[a],*, Erin A. Gillaspie, MD, MPH[b,1]

KEYWORDS

- Traumatic diaphragm injury • Diaphragm hernia • Diaphragm rupture • Thoracoabdominal trauma

KEY POINTS

- Diaphragm injuries are rare and difficult to diagnose.
- Clinicians should have a high index of suspicion when a traumatic mechanism is suggestive of diaphragm injury.
- When identified, diaphragm injuries should be repaired.
- Delayed diagnosis of diaphragm injuries may carry high morbidity and risk of mortality.

INTRODUCTION

Traumatic diaphragm injury (TDI) is rare, accounting for only 1% of all traumatic injuries,[1] and occurs in 0.8% to 15% of all trauma patients.[2–5] The diaphragm can sustain a direct laceration secondary to a penetrating trauma or rupture due to blunt trauma.[6] The mechanism of blunt traumatic rupture is postulated to be from an increased trans-diaphragmatic pressure gradient in the setting of anterior thoracoabdominal trauma. A second mechanism is a shearing or avulsion injury with tearing of the lateral attachments seen in lateral impact blunt trauma.[1–3,6–8] The majority of patients with a diaphragm injury have associated injuries,[5] and a higher injury severity score.[9]

Blunt Traumatic Diaphragm Rupture

Blunt traumatic diaphragm rupture occurs in 0.8% to 1.6% of all blunt trauma patients,[5] and in 1% to 7% of patients sustaining blunt thoracoabdominal trauma.[2,3] The most common traumatic mechanisms resulting in diaphragm injury are high speed motor vehicle collision, fall from height, and crush injuries.[10]

Diaphragm rupture is more common on the left side compared to the right, due to the protective effect of the liver.[3,5,8,10] Injuries to the right hemidiaphragm require higher force resulting in higher rate of pre-hospital mortality.[11] Injuries on the left side will most commonly occur in the posterolateral aspect of the diaphragm which is derived from the pleuroperitoneal membrane and is the weakest portion of the diaphragm structurally, or at the central tendon (additional anatomic details described in Chapter 1).[3,7,8,11] Blunt TDI tends to result in larger injuries than penetrating trauma.[12]

As noted earlier, patients generally present with associated injuries, and thus carry a high mortality rate (15%–32%).[13]

Penetrating Traumatic Diaphragm Injuries

Diaphragm injury is diagnosed in 10% to 15% of patients presenting with penetrating thoracoabdominal trauma.[3] While there are regional variances in blunt to penetrating trauma ratios, nationally penetrating traumas account for approximately 66% to 67% of TDIs.[14,15] Penetrating injuries are typically smaller than blunt ruptures or avulsion injuries and are therefore more difficult to diagnose[3,12] therefore, the actual incidence is unknown.[3] Additionally, with increasing selective non-operative management, these smaller injuries

[a] Division of Acute Care Surgery, Department of Surgery, University of Tennessee Medical Center Knoxville, 1924 Alcoa Highway Box U-11, Knoxville, TN 37920, USA; [b] Division of thoracic Surgery, Creighton University Medical Center CHI Health, 7500 Mercy Road, Omaha, NE 68124, USA
[1] Present address: 7500 Mercy Road, Omaha, NE 68124.
* Corresponding author.
E-mail address: dgillaspie@utmck.edu

Thorac Surg Clin 34 (2024) 171–178
https://doi.org/10.1016/j.thorsurg.2024.01.008

without obvious computed tomography findings go undiagnosed.[14]

Delayed Diaphragm Injury

Delayed manifestation, days after index injury, may occur in the setting of devitalization of tissue or ischemia and ultimately weakening and rupture of the diaphragm.[6,16] This could cause injury to be missed on imaging as it looks often like inflammation, and even under direct visualization during operative exploration.[6]

Missed Injuries

Up to 70% of diaphragm injuries may be missed in the acute setting, and as many as 18% missed at time of laparotomy.[10,17,18]

Missed injuries may present later with herniation of abdominal contents into the chest. While in some cases, patients may be asymptomatic, others may have shortness of breath, chest pain, abdominal pain, or obstructive symptoms.[1,10,17] While rare, patients may develop gastric outlet obstruction, small bowel, or even large bowel obstruction.[10,19–22]

Time from injury to presentation is widely variable, ranging from 2 months with some reported findings as far out as 50 years from injury.[1,21]

Blunt injuries tend to be larger and thus have a higher rate of long-term complications comparatively.[12] However, even small penetrating injuries can enlarge over time and negative pleural pressures create a gradient that facilitate herniation of abdominal contents into the thorax.[1,13,19,21]

The risk of missed injury includes incarceration and strangulation of viscera.[3,19] Morbidity associated with missed diaphragm injury is approximately 30%, and the overall mortality rate is 10% to 25%.[5,20] Mortality associated with strangulated viscera can be as high as 80% to 85%.[10,20]

DIAGNOSIS & MANAGEMENT

Diagnosis of TDI can be challenging, accounting for the number of missed injuries and delayed presentations.[1,4] A high index of suspicion must be maintained—the mechanism of injury as well as pattern of injuries serve as important clues. As noted previously, a history of high velocity crash, fall from height, direct abdominal blunt force injury, or penetrating injury in the upper abdomen or low chest should prompt consideration of a diaphragm injury. A clinical examination contributes very little to the diagnosis.

Imaging is an important diagnostic tool, particularly in stable patients.[3] Traumatic diaphragm injuries are accurately identified on fewer than 50% of plain film chest X-rays with a sensitivity between 27% and 68% for left side injuries, and as low as 17% to 33% for identification of right side TDI.[1,5,23] Sensitivity improves to 94% when there is herniation of abdominal contents into the thorax.[24] Interpretation of chest X-ray is another limitation. In a trauma setting, the accuracy of identification of a TDI by the trauma leader is only 22%.[24]

The increasing availability and common use of computed tomography (CT) scans has improved identification of TDI. CT scans of the chest, abdomen, and pelvis have a diagnostic sensitivity of 87% and specificity of 72%.[3] Sensitivity is higher for left-sided injuries compared to right and the right also has higher rates of delayed diagnosis likely due to the liver and diaphragm sharing similar contrast enhancement and the lack of intervening fat.[1,3,5,13] CT does carry a false-positive rate most commonly attributable to chronic congenital or acquired hernias or eventration/paralysis of the diaphragm.[23]

Findings on Computed Tomography

The classic CT signs suggestive of diaphragm injury are the discontinuous diaphragm sign, dependent viscera sign, herniation of viscera into the thoracic cavity, dangling diaphragm sign, a wound tract through the diaphragm, hump sign, collar sign, and band sign.[5,8,10,19,25–27] These can be divided into direct and indirect signs summarized in **Table 1**.[10]

DIRECT SIGNS

Diaphragmatic discontinuity on CT presents as a non-visualized segment of diaphragm representing the site of injury (**Fig. 1**). The free edges may be thickened and demarcate the extent of the defect.[10] This is seen more often in blunt trauma, and has a sensitivity of 36% to 82% and specifitity of 88% to 95%.[10]

The dangling diaphragm sign is generally best seen on a coronal or sagittal reconstruction of the CT scan and is the curling of the torn edge of the diaphragm toward the abdomen (**Fig. 2**). This is frequently described to be in the shape of a "comma."[10,25] The sensitivity and specificity of the dangling diaphragm sign is 54% and 98%, respectively.[10]

INDIRECT SIGNS

The dependent viscera sign manifests on a CT with the patient in supine position. Herniated abdominal contents may be seen in direct apposition to the posterior chest wall—on the right the liver is

Table 1
Computed tomography signs and finding of diaphragmatic injury

Sign	Imaging Findings
Discontinuous diaphragm sign	Segmental non-visualization of the diaphragm
Diaphragm thickening	Comparative thickening of the diaphragm at a site of injury, there may or may not be evidence of retraction of the edges
Dependent viscera sign	Right side: when the upper third of the liver abuts the posterior ribs on the right Left side: when the stomach or bowel abuts the posterior ribs or lay posterior to the spleen on the left
Herniation of viscera into the chest	The presence of intra-abdominal organs within the thoracic cavity through a defect in the diaphragm
Dangling diaphragm sign	The free edge of the diaphragm (torn edge) curls inward from its normal course, usually at right angles to the chest wall (comma shape)
Wound track trajectory/ contiguous injury	In a penetrating trauma, the identification of contiguous injuries above and below the diaphragm implies injury of the diaphragm as well. The wound track can be traced through the diaphragm.
Collar sign	Waist-like narrowing of the abdominal viscus at the torn level of the diaphragm.
Hump sign	This variation of the collar sign occurs on the right when a rounded segment of the liver protruding through the diaphragm injury forming a "hump"-shaped mass
Band sign	Another variation on the collar sign, described as a linear lucency across the liver along the torn edge of the diaphragm

Adapted from Panda A, Kumar A, Gamanagatti S, Patil A, Kumar S, Gupta A. Traumatic diaphragmatic injury: a review of CT signs and the difference between blunt and penetrating injury. Diagn Interv Radiol. 2014;20(2):121-8. https://doi.org/10.5152/dir.2013.13248.

directly overlying the posterior thorax or ribs and on the left the stomach or small bowel is seen in contact with the posterior thorax or posterior to the spleen.[8,10,25] This sign is identified most commonly with posterior diaphragm injuries.[8,10]

Herniation of abdominal contents has a high specificity of 94% to 100% but sensitivity drops to 8% to 81% because signs of right-sided liver herniation are more subtle.[10] Additional radiographic criteria that help to facilitate the diagnosis

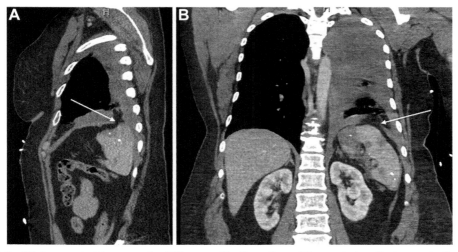

Fig. 1. (*A*) Sagittal computed tomography (CT) scan with disruption of the posterior diaphragm indicated by arrow and concomitant hemothorax. (*B*) Coronal representation of the same patient with diaphragmatic defect indicated by the arrow.

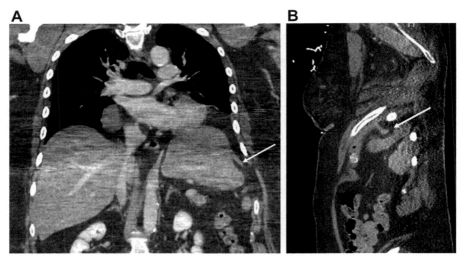

Fig. 2. Coronal (*A*) and sagittal (*B*) CT scan demonstrating a dangling diaphragm sign with an arrow denoting the curling edge of the diaphragm.

are the collar sign, hump sign, and band sign. The Collar sign is the luminal narrowing of herniated viscera as it traverses the diaphragm creating the appearance of a waist on imaging **(Fig. 3)**.[8,10,25] The hump sign and band sign are unique to the right side. The hump sign is the rounded or hump-like appearance of a small portion of liver that has herniated through a diaphragm defect.[8,25] The band sign is linear lucency or bright line that intersects the liver at the level of the torn diaphragm indicating

impingement or compromised perfusion from the pressure of the diaphragm.[8,25]

A contiguous injury is represented by 2 injuries that are continuous with one another arising on both sides of the hemidiaphragm (**Fig. 4**); these can generally be traced through a common track with the interceding diaphragm. While a direct diaphragm injury may not be visible, it is suggested by the trajectory of the wound and surrounding damage.[25] This is more commonly seen in penetrating trauma.[25]

Retrospective review of imaging after a confirmed injury has identified the discontinuous diaphragm sign and diaphragm thickening as the 2 most common findings on CT.[25] The dependent viscera sign and collar sign were only identified in patients who had sustained blunt trauma. A dangling diaphragm was found in both blunt and penetrating, but more common in the former and a contiguous injury was seen exclusively in penetrating trauma.[19,25] The CT finding of any of these signs is highly specific and help to rule in an injury; however, the absence of such a sign does not rule out injury.[26]

Laparoscopy for Identification of Diaphragm Injuries

The role of laparoscopy in trauma has been debated for decades. In general, it has no role in critical or unstable patients. Contemporarily, as in other types of injuries, the role of laparoscopy in the diagnosis and management of diaphragm injuries has been investigated in stable patients.[20,21,28–34] Outcomes vary by study and the indications for laparoscopic assessment lack consensus. For patients with thoracoabdominal penetrating injuries, The Eastern Association for

Fig. 3. Coronal CT scan demonstrating herniation of the stomach through the diaphragm and the classic collar sign with luminal narrowing of the stomach.

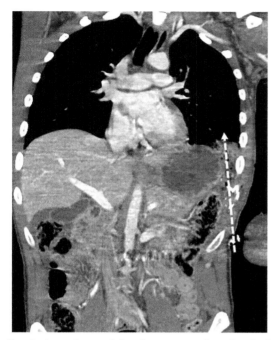

Fig. 4. A contiguous injury has no overt imaging findings that clearly demonstrate diaphragmatic involvement of an injury. The injury is inferred by a continuous path, generally a penetrating injury, involving structures above and below the diaphragm. Here, you can see and injury to the eighth rib on the left, fluid and air within the abdomen adjacent tto the stomach, and additional air and fluid in the costodiaphragmatic recess. The trajectory of the ballistic is demonstrated with the *dotted line*.

the Surgery of Trauma (EAST) conditionally recommends diagnostic laparoscopy to avoid a missed diaphragm injury in patients who are stable with no other indication for surgery where the trajectory raises suspicion for occult diaphragm injury.[14] There is some data to recommend CT-first approach to these stable patients, looking for CT-findings such as contiguous injury on either side of the diaphragm, and other signs that are suggestive of injury.[14]

Considerations must balance likelihood of injury with concomitant injuries. In a patient with penetrating trauma, no other sites of injury, and high suspicion of diaphragmatic injury, a diagnostic laparoscopy can be performed safely and serve as a valuable tool in detecting occult injuries.[34] Unfortunately, while some experts advocate for diagnostic utility of laparoscopy as a routine tool to rule in or out diaphragmatic injury, this has been shown to have a high negative laparoscopy rate (75%) thus exposing patient to added risk and cost without benefit.[21,30,35,36] Further, while diagnostic laparoscopy has been found adequate to diagnose and

treat isolated diaphragm injuries,[29] it is less reliable in detecting hollow viscus injuries, and should be reserved for patients in whom laparotomy is not indicated.[37]

In both penetrating and blunt trauma, if a diaphragm injury is identified, no additional injuries exist, and the patient is hemodynamically stable, a laparoscopic approach to repair is safe.[28] Further, when comparing laparoscopy versus laparotomy for repair of diaphragm injury, it was found that patients undergoing laparoscopy had a lower morbidity and shorter length of stay compared with laparotomy.[35] EAST in their latest practice management guidelines conditionally recommended laparoscopic approach over laparotomy for repair of isolated diaphragm injuries.[14]

Video-Assisted Thoracoscopic Surgery

In penetrating thoracoabdominal traumas, the role of thoracoscopy has been investigated in patients who presented with normal vital signs, no other signs of injury requiring emergent operation, and were found on chest X-ray to have a hemothorax and/or pneumothorax.[38,39]

Penetrating trauma causing diaphragm injury was most often at the seventh, eightth, and ninth intercostal spaces.[38] Thoracoscopy was found to be a reliable tool for the identification and management of occult diaphragm injuries,[3,38–41] with a sensitivity of close to 100%.[3] Importantly, if a concomitant abdominal injury is suspected, an abdominal exploration is required in addition to thoracoscopy.[38] For right-sided injuries, a combined thoracoscopic and laparoscopic approach has been described in the absence of additional injury, simply to enhance visualization of the right diaphragm which is more difficult to evaluate from the abdominal approach.[42]

EAST does not specifically comment on thoracoscopy in their latest practice management guidelines but acknowledges that there are studies that describe better visibility and diagnostic accuracy of video-assisted thoracoscopic surgery (VATS) when compared with laparoscopy, particularly in posterior and right-sided injuries.[14] They do, however, recommend routine abdominal evaluation if a diaphragm injury is found to directly rule out intra-abdominal injury.[14] For a stable patient with a diaphragm injury, EAST recommends an abdominal approach as preferable over a thoracic approach in the acute setting.[14]

Management

The management of a diaphragm injury is impacted by the presentation and associated injuries. Ideally all diaphragm injuries are repaired in an acute setting as there is a low likelihood of spontaneous healing both secondary to the continuous diaphragmatic movement and pressure gradient between the thoracic and abdominal cavity facilitating enlargement and herniation of intraabdominal contents over time.[41] In addition, when left untreated, patients face the potential for future morbidity and mortality.[7,17]

The surgical approach to the diaphragm is largely dictated by the presence of associated injuries and adequacy of exposure, and a dual approach can be very useful.

Patients with chest injury manifesting with a hemothorax or pneumothorax on imaging may undergo a VATS exploration with repair of diaphragm injury. Published experiences describe safe, efficient, and effective treatment of the diaphragm through a thoracoscopic approach.[38,40]

Likewise, laparoscopy, laparotomy, and even a thoracoabdominal approach have been described each with inherent benefits allowing the diaphragm and additional injuries to be efficaciously addressed.

The surgical tenets of repair of a diaphragmatic trauma are the same regardless of the approach. First, associated injuries must be addressed. It should be noted that to facilitate optimal access to the abdomen, in most cases, patients will be in supine position. While this is ideal for an anterior diaphragmatic injury, it may impede visualization of a more posterior injury and make repair difficult. The diaphragm and injury must be fully visualized. Devitalized tissue should be debrided. If a primary closure is possible, the diaphragm is reapproximated with non-absorbable sutures in either an interrupted, figure-of-eight, or horizontal mattress fashion most commonly taking full thickness bites.[3,7,41,43] Pledgets may be employed to reduce tearing of the muscle. Closure should ideally be tension free; however, for closures under significant tension or for large destructive injuries, mesh may be required.[27,43,44] If there is a hollow viscus perforation, the thoracic and abdominal cavities should be vigorously irrigated and drains placed.[41]

Delayed presentation of chronic diaphragm injuries also require repair. In an asymptomatic or minimally symptomatic patient, this may be accomplished electively; however, for those presenting with strangulation, they must be cared for emergently.[41] The surgical approach in the chronic setting should take into consideration presenting clinical scenario, surgeon preference and experience, prior abdominal surgery with scarring, and likelihood of adhesions within the chest that would not be safely addressed from an abdominal vantage. A minimally invasive approach may be considered for stable patients.[7]

Complications of both acute and chronic repair include dehiscence of repair, recurrent herniation, iatrogenic injury to the phrenic nerve, subdiaphragmatic abscess, empyema, and respiratory insufficiency.[45] A unique risk related to the repair of a chronic diaphragm injury with herniation is abdominal compartment syndrome after reduction of the intrathoracic contents.

DISCUSSION

Traumatic diaphragm injury is seen in 0.8% to 15% of all trauma patients, with increasing incidence due to increased rate of high velocity blunt trauma from motor vehicle collisions.[5] Traumatic diaphragm injuries can be difficult to diagnose, and missed injuries may manifest later as large defects, herniation of abdominal viscera, and in some cases, life-threatening strangulation of content.[10,19,20]

Clinical symptoms are non-specific and may include chest pain, abdominal pain, dyspnea, or orthopnea.[7] Chest X-ray (CXR) is unreliable for diagnosis in the acute setting. With more readily available and the ability to perform a CT rapidly, this has supplanted the use of CXR for diagnosis and has a sensitivity and specificity above 80%.[46] CT findings supporting a diagnosis of diaphragmatic injury include discontinuous diaphragm sign, dependent viscera sign, herniation of viscera into the thoracic cavity, dangling diaphragm sign, wound tract through the diaphragm, hump sign, collar sign, and band sign.[5,8,10,19,25–27]

Historically, exploration was considered mandatory for penetrating thoracoabdominal trauma, and rates of negative laparotomy were 40% and morbidity rates were high.[44] With the increased rates of non-operative management of both penetrating and blunt trauma, the rate of missed diaphragm injury has also increased.[3,38]

Presenting clinical scenarios and associated injuries should raise suspicion for diaphragm injury. The most common associated injuries are pelvic fractures, rib fractures, intraperitoneal hemorrhage, liver laceration, splenic laceration, pneumothorax, pulmonary contusions, intrapleural bleeding, and injury to the thoracic aorta.[8,47–49]

TDI should ideally be repaired at the time of diagnosis, accounting for patient stability and other injuries.[17] Prognosis related to a diaphragm injury is good if repaired promptly, delay in diagnosis is associated with increased morbidity and mortality.[3] The surgical approach should be tailored to the patient and presentation and may include thoracoscopy, laparoscopy, laparotomy, or combined thoraco-abdominal. A primary repair is feasible in most cases.

SUMMARY

Suspicion for TDI should be maintained with patients presenting with penetrating or high-velocity blunt trauma to the thoracoabdominal region. In stable patients, CT scan should be considered. If there is no other indication for operative intervention and clinical suspicion is high, laparoscopy or thoracoscopy should be considered to evaluate for occult injury.

CLINICS CARE POINTS

- Clinical symptoms of diaphragm injury are non-specific and may include chest pain, abdominal pain, dyspnea, orthopnea
- Sensitivity and specificity of CT is better than chest X-Ray
- When diagnosed, diaphragm injuries should be repaired, both in the acute and delayed settings
- Missed injuries can result in delayed presentation, with increased morbidity and mortality.

DISCLOSURE

D. Gillaspie authors have nothing to disclose. E.A. Gillaspie serves on advisory boards for Genentech, AstraZeneca and BMS. She is a speaker for BMS. None are pertinent to this article.

REFERENCES

1. Alsuwayj AH, Al Nasser AH, Al Dehailan AM, et al. Giant Traumatic Diaphragmatic Hernia: A Report of Delayed Presentation. Cureus 2021;13(12):e20315.
2. Berg RJ, Okoye O, Teixeira PG, et al. The double jeopardy of blunt thoracoabdominal trauma. Arch Surg 2012;147(6):498–504.
3. Cardoso LF, Gonçalves MVC, Machado CJ, et al. Retrospective analysis of 103 diaphragmatic injuries in patients operated in a trauma center. Rev Col Bras Cir 2017;44(3):245–51.
4. Athanassiadi K, Kalavrouziotis G, Athanassiou M, et al. Blunt diaphragmatic rupture. Eur J Cardio Thorac Surg 1999;15(4):469–74.
5. Baldwin M, Dagens A, Sgromo B. Laparoscopic management of a delayed traumatic diaphragmatic rupture complicated by bowel strangulation. J Surg Case Rep 2014;2014(7). https://doi.org/10.1093/jscr/rju073.
6. Hamidian Jahromi A, Pennywell D, Owings JT. Does a Negative Emergency Celiotomy Exclude the Possibility of Significant Diaphragmatic Injury? A Case Report and Review of the Literature. Trauma Mon 2016;21(4):e25053.
7. Gielis M, Bruera N, Pinsak A, et al. Laparoscopic repair of acute traumatic diaphragmatic hernia with mesh reinforcement: A case report. Int J Surg Case Rep 2022;93:106910.
8. Gmachowska A, Pacho R, Anysz-Grodzicka A, et al. The Role of Computed Tomography in the Diagnostics of Diaphragmatic Injury After Blunt Thoraco-Abdominal Trauma. Pol J Radiol 2016;81:522–8.
9. Schurr LA, Thiedemann C, Alt V, et al. Diaphragmatic Injuries among Severely Injured Patients (ISS ≥ 16)-An Indicator of Injury Pattern and Severity of Abdominal Trauma. Medicina (Kaunas). 2022; 58(11). https://doi.org/10.3390/medicina58111596.
10. Kaur R, Prabhakar A, Kochhar S, et al. Blunt traumatic diaphragmatic hernia: Pictorial review of CT signs. Indian J Radiol Imaging 2015;25(3):226–32.
11. Petrone P, Asensio JA, Marini CP. Diaphragmatic injuries and post-traumatic diaphragmatic hernias. Curr Probl Surg 2017;54(1):11–32.
12. Abdellatif W, Chow B, Hamid S, et al. Unravelling the Mysteries of Traumatic Diaphragmatic Injury: An Up-to-Date Review. Can Assoc Radiol J 2020;71(3): 313–21.
13. Hogarty J, Jassal K, Ravintharan N, et al. Twenty-year perspective on blunt traumatic diaphragmatic injury in level 1 trauma centre: Early versus delayed diagnosis injury patterns and outcomes. Emerg Med Australas 2023. https://doi.org/10.1111/1742-6723.14255.
14. McDonald AA, Robinson BRH, Alarcon L, et al. Evaluation and management of traumatic diaphragmatic injuries: A Practice Management Guideline from the Eastern Association for the Surgery of Trauma. J Trauma Acute Care Surg 2018;85(1):198–207.
15. van Wyk C, Hlaise KK, Blumenthal R. Traumatic Diaphragmatic Injuries at Medicolegal Autopsy: A 1-Year Prospective Study. Am J Forensic Med Pathol 2022;43(4):347–53.
16. Rashid F, Chakrabarty MM, Singh R, et al. A review on delayed presentation of diaphragmatic rupture. World J Emerg Surg 2009;4:32.
17. Zhao L, Han Z, Liu H, et al. Delayed traumatic diaphragmatic rupture: diagnosis and surgical treatment. J Thorac Dis 2019;11(7):2774–7.
18. Malherbe GF, Navsaria PH, Nicol AJ, et al. Laparoscopy or clinical follow-up to detect occult diaphragm injuries following left-sided thoracoabdominal stab wounds: A pilot randomized controlled trial. S Afr J Surg 2017;55(4):20–5.
19. Hammer MM, Flagg E, Mellnick VM, et al. Computed tomography of blunt and penetrating diaphragmatic injury: sensitivity and inter-observer agreement of CT Signs. Emerg Radiol 2014;21(2):143–9.
20. D'Souza N, Clarke D, Laing G. Prevalence, management and outcome of traumatic diaphragm injuries managed by the Pietermaritzburg Metropolitan Trauma Service. Ann R Coll Surg Engl 2017;99(5): 394–401.

21. Chern TY, Kwok A, Putnis S. A case of tension faecop-neumothorax after delayed diagnosis of traumatic diaphragmatic hernia. Surg Case Rep 2018;4(1):37.

22. Bhatti UH, Dawani S. Large bowel obstruction complicating a posttraumatic diaphragmatic hernia. Singapore Med J 2015;56(4):e56–8.

23. Leung VA, Patlas MN, Reid S, et al. Imaging of Traumatic Diaphragmatic Rupture: Evaluation of Diagnostic Accuracy at a Level 1 Trauma Centre. Can Assoc Radiol J 2015;66(4):310–7.

24. Hanna WC, Ferri LE, Fata P, et al. The current status of traumatic diaphragmatic injury: lessons learned from 105 patients over 13 years. Ann Thorac Surg 2008;85(3):1044–8.

25. Panda A, Kumar A, Gamanagatti S, et al. Traumatic diaphragmatic injury: a review of CT signs and the difference between blunt and penetrating injury. Diagn Interv Radiol 2014;20(2):121–8.

26. Dreizin D, Bergquist PJ, Taner AT, et al. Evolving concepts in MDCT diagnosis of penetrating diaphragmatic injury. Emerg Radiol 2015;22(2):149–56.

27. Gao JM, Du DY, Li H, et al. Traumatic diaphragmatic rupture with combined thoracoabdominal injuries: Difference between penetrating and blunt injuries. Chin J Traumatol 2015;18(1):21–6.

28. Campos Costa F, Cardoso V, Monteiro AM, et al. Laparoscopic Repair of an Acute Traumatic Diaphragmatic Hernia: Clinical Case. Cureus 2020; 12(10):e11082.

29. Friese RS, Coln CE, Gentilello LM. Laparoscopy is sufficient to exclude occult diaphragm injury after penetrating abdominal trauma. J Trauma 2005; 58(4):789–92.

30. Murray JA, Demetriades D, Asensio JA, et al. Occult injuries to the diaphragm: prospective evaluation of laparoscopy in penetrating injuries to the left lower chest. J Am Coll Surg 1998;187(6):626–30.

31. Zantut LF, Ivatury RR, Smith RS, et al. Diagnostic and therapeutic laparoscopy for penetrating abdominal trauma: a multicenter experience. J Trauma 1997;42(5):825–9 [discussion: 829–31].

32. Zafar SN, Onwugbufor MT, Hughes K, et al. Laparoscopic surgery for trauma: the realm of therapeutic management. Am J Surg 2015;209(4):627–32.

33. Yucel T, Gonullu D, Matur R, et al. Laparoscopic management of left thoracoabdominal stab wounds: a prospective study. Surg Laparosc Endosc Percutan Tech 2010;20(1):42–5.

34. Powell BS, Magnotti LJ, Schroeppel TJ, et al. Diagnostic laparoscopy for the evaluation of occult diaphragmatic injury following penetrating thoracoabdominal trauma. Injury 2008;39(5):530–4.

35. Obaid O, Hammad A, Bible L, et al. Open Versus Laparoscopic Repair of Traumatic Diaphragmatic Injury: A Nationwide Propensity-Matched Analysis. J Surg Res 2021;268:452–8.

36. D'Souza N, Bruce JL, Clarke DL, et al. Laparoscopy for Occult Left-sided Diaphragm Injury Following Penetrating Thoracoabdominal Trauma is Both Diagnostic and Therapeutic. Surg Laparosc Endosc Percutan Tech 2016;26(1):e5–8.

37. O'Malley E, Boyle E, O'Callaghan A, et al. Role of laparoscopy in penetrating abdominal trauma: a systematic review. World J Surg 2013;37(1):113–22.

38. Bagheri R, Tavassoli A, Sadrizadeh A, et al. The role of thoracoscopy for the diagnosis of hidden diaphragmatic injuries in penetrating thoracoabdominal trauma. Interact Cardiovasc Thorac Surg 2009;9(2): 195–7 [discussion: 197–8].

39. Freeman RK, Al-Dossari G, Hutcheson KA, et al. Indications for using video-assisted thoracoscopic surgery to diagnose diaphragmatic injuries after penetrating chest trauma. Ann Thorac Surg 2001; 72(2):342–7.

40. Martinez M, Briz JE, Carillo EH. Video thoracoscopy expedites the diagnosis and treatment of penetrating diaphragmatic injuries. Surg Endosc 2001; 15(1):28–32 [discussion: 33].

41. Furák J, Athanassiadi K. Diaphragm and transdiaphragmatic injuries. J Thorac Dis 2019;11(Suppl 2):S152–7.

42. Shichiri K, Imamura K, Takada M, et al. Minimally invasive repair of right-sided blunt traumatic diaphragmatic injury. BMJ Case Rep 2020;13(11). https://doi.org/10.1136/bcr-2020-235870.

43. Shaban Y, Elkbuli A, McKenney M, et al. Traumatic Diaphragmatic Rupture with Transthoracic Organ Herniation: A Case Report and Review of Literature. Am J Case Rep 2020;21:e919442.

44. Tserng TL, Gatmaitan MB. Laparoscopic approach to the management of penetrating traumatic diaphragmatic injury. Trauma Case Rep 2017;10:4–11.

45. Conti L, Grassi C, Delfanti R, et al. Left diaphragmatic rupture in vehicle trauma: Report of surgical treatment and complications of two consecutive cases. Acta Biomed 2021;92(S1):e2021121.

46. Yucel M, Bas G, Kulalı F, et al. Evaluation of diaphragm in penetrating left thoracoabdominal stab injuries: The role of multislice computed tomography. Injury 2015;46(9):1734–7.

47. Hofmann S, Kornmann M, Henne-Bruns D, et al. Traumatic diaphragmatic ruptures: clinical presentation, diagnosis and surgical approach in adults. GMS Interdiscip Plast Reconstr Surg DGPW 2012; 1:Doc02.

48. Lim KH, Park J. Blunt traumatic diaphragmatic rupture: Single-center experience with 38 patients. Medicine (Baltim) 2018;97(41):e12849.

49. Lim BL, Teo LT, Chiu MT, et al. Traumatic diaphragmatic injuries: a retrospective review of a 12-year experience at a tertiary trauma centre. Singapore Med J 2017;58(10):595–600.

Management of Diaphragm Paralysis and Eventration

Camille Yongue, MD[a], Travis C. Geraci, MD[a],
Stephanie H. Chang, MD, MSCI[a],*

KEYWORDS

- Eventration • Diaphragm paralysis • Diaphragm plication • Phrenic nerve paralysis
- Phrenic nerve injury

KEY POINTS

- Diaphragm paralysis is an acquired condition resulting in elevation of the diaphragm due to disruption or dysfunction of the phrenic nerve.
- Most patients are asymptomatic and may not require surgery, though patients with symptomatic diaphgram elevations are candidates for surgical repair.
- Improvement in lung volume with flattening of the diaphragm is the primary goal of diaphragm plication.
- Minimally invasive thoracoscopic diaphragm plication is safe and has excellent outcomes.

INTRODUCTION

The diaphragm is a muscle that is essential for normal pulmonary respiration. The diaphragm is composed of skeletal muscle that inserts onto a central tendon, separating the thoracic and abdominal cavities. Two hemidiaphragms—left and right—work simultaneously for optimal pulmonary function.[1] Diaphragm dysfunction often presents as an elevated hemidiaphragm, which can be unilateral or bilateral. A dysfunctional diaphragm can be classified as either diaphragm eventration or paralysis. The exact incidence of diaphragm impairment is unknown due to its asymptomatic nature in the majority of patients. However, some patients with diaphragm dysfunction can have significant respiratory impairment such as hypoventilation, hypoxia, and atelectasis.[2]

Eventration of the diaphragm occurs when part or all of the diaphragm is elevated due to decreased muscle fibers,[3] with abdominal organs displacing the diaphragm superiorly. Eventration can be congenital but most frequently occurs with increasing age. Idiopathic eventration is not uncommon, with one study demonstrating that no etiology was identified in 57% of reported cases of diaphragm elevation.[4] The presentation and management of congenital diaphragm eventration will not be covered in this article.

Diaphragm paralysis is an acquired condition resulting in elevation of one or both hemidiaphragms due to phrenic nerve injury or dysfunction. The phrenic nerve arises from the third to fifth cervical nerves courses through the neck anterior to the scalene muscles, descends along the mediastinum anteromedially to the pulmonary hilum and then parallels the pericardiophrenic branch of the internal mammary artery (IMA), and inserts onto the diaphragm (IMA). On the left, the phrenic crosses the IMA from lateral to medial then runs along the pericardium to the diaphragm. On the right, the phrenic runs along the right brachiocephalic vein, superior vena cava, pericardium of the right atrium, and inferior vena cava. Trauma from either non-iatrogenic causes (motor vehicle accident) or iatrogenic causes (surgery) can affect

[a] Department of Cardiothoracic Surgery, Division of Thoracic Surgery, New York University Langone Health, 530 First Avenue, Suite 9V, New York, NY 10016, USA
* Corresponding author.
E-mail address: stephanie.chang@nyulangone.org

Thorac Surg Clin 34 (2024) 179–187
https://doi.org/10.1016/j.thorsurg.2024.01.006
1547-4127/24/© 2024 Elsevier Inc. All rights reserved.

the nerve at any point along its course and can cause mechanical disruption. Disruption of the nerve results in lack of innervation to the diaphragm with resultant atrophy of the muscle.

PRESENTATION OF DIAPHRAGM DYSFUNCTION

Presentation of diaphragm eventration or paralysis can vary widely. Frequently, an elevated hemidiaphragm is asymptomatic and incidentally noted on imaging. The most common symptom associated with hemidiaphragm elevation is dyspnea caused by impaired ventilation and manifested with a ventilation–perfusion mismatch at the lung bases. Decreased lung volumes can also cause restrictive symptoms and moderate hypoxemia, which is worse when lying supine.[2] Orthopnea is another common symptom, resulting from abdominal contents pressing upward on the diaphragm when supine.

DIAGNOSIS OF DIAPHRAGM DYSFUNCTION

Proper evaluation of an incidentally discovered elevated hemidiaphragm includes diagnostic testing and pulmonary function testing (PFT), to determine the etiology.

Diagnostic Testing

Chest Radiograph: Diaphragm elevation is often discovered incidentally on chest radiograph (CXR). In patients with normal diaphragm function, the dome of the right diaphragm projects over the anterior 5th to 6th rib and the posterior 10th rib. The left hemidiaphragm is naturally lower than the right by one interspace on average (**Fig. 1**A).[5] Both partial and total eventration can be identified on CXR, most commonly in the anteromedial portion of the right hemidiaphragm. Total eventration will appear identical to hemidiaphragm paralysis, though in hemidiaphragm paralysis there will often be an adjacent area of atelectatic lung due to lack of movement. Diaphragm paralysis can appear on CXR as an accentuated dome with deepened costophrenic angles (**Fig. 1**B).

Fluoroscopy: The "sniff test" is the gold standard to determine whether there is phrenic nerve involvement in cases of diaphragm elevation found on imaging. The sniff test is a fluoroscopic examination typically performed with the patient upright, though supine positioning removes the gravitational aid to the diaphragm. The patient is instructed to inhale rapidly and forcefully through the nose with the mouth closed. In a normal sniff test, a brief rapid descent of the diaphragm bilaterally will be seen under fluoroscopy (**Fig. 2**A, B). Normal diaphragm excursion is between 3 and 5 cm. An abnormal sniff test is the paradoxic motion of a hemidiaphragm upward by greater than 2 cm which can indicate diaphragm paralysis (**Fig. 3**A, B). The sniff test is positive in 90% of patients with unilateral phrenic nerve palsy. In bilateral paralysis, both hemidiaphragms move upward on inspiration and passively downward on expiration.

The sniff test can also detect diaphragm weakness or eventration. Chronic obstructive pulmonary disease, severe weakness due to prolonged ventilatory support, or diaphragm eventration will lead to limited diaphragm excursion on inhalation. However, there is minimal excursion of the diaphragm without paradoxic motion, which differentiates it from paralysis.

Ultrasound: Ultrasound can also be used to evaluate paradoxic motion via sniff test, similar to fluoroscopy. The limitations of this approach include the small field of view, possible difficulty visualizing the left hemidiaphragm due to gaseous distention or obesity, and it depends on operator skill.

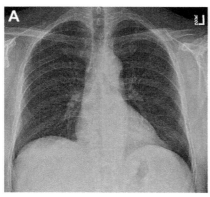
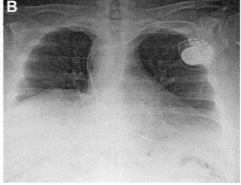

Fig. 1. (*A*) Normal chest radiograph with the right hemidiaphragm slightly elevated compared with the left. (*B*) Abnormal chest radiography with significantly elevated right hemidiaphragm.

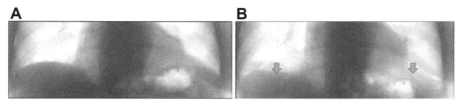

Fig. 2. Fluoroscopy demonstrating a normal sniff test. (*A*) The hemidiaphragms are equal levels at rest. (*B*) Both hemidiaphragms have downward excursion (shown with *blue arrows*) with inspiration.

Computed tomography scan: A standard chest computed tomography (CT) can demonstrate an elevated hemidiaphragm as well as assess for underlying causes such as malignancy or aneurysms, leading to phrenic nerve dysfunction.[6] Owing to the variety of possible underlying causes, a chest CT should be routinely performed for the workup of an elevated hemidiaphragm. Dynamic chest CT can be performed but is often of limited use.

Electromyography: Electromyography can be used to determine whether there is phrenic nerve paralysis by using direct nerve stimulation; however, this is not routinely obtained.

Pulmonary Function Testing

All patients undergoing evaluation for an elevated hemidiaphragm should have PFT in upright and supine positions to determine the impact of diaphragm elevation on respiration and identify any confounding respiratory processes. Impairment in diaphragm function can lead to reductions in vital capacity, total lung capacity, and tidal volume leading to reduced functional residual capacity.[7] PFT may reveal a restrictive pattern with a 20% to 50% reduction in total lung capacity when the patient is supine.[8]

Etiology

Diaphragm eventration in adults is either a congenital condition that is discovered when the patient is an adult or slowly acquired due to advanced age with decreased muscle fibers. As patients age, decreased muscle fibers in the setting of increased abdominal pressure (such as with obesity) leads to progressive elevation of the affected diaphragm. If a sniff test demonstrates limited excursion with no paradoxic motion, without underlying parenchymal lung disease such as idiopathic pulmonary fibrosis, then the elevated diaphragm is secondary to eventration.

If the sniff test confirms diaphragmatic paralysis, then the mechanism of underlying phrenic nerve dysfunction should be delineated. In some situations, diaphragm paralysis may be reversible, often

secondary to iatrogenic injury of the nerve. For patients who undergo cardiac surgery, damage due to hypothermia from cold topical cardioplegia or ice near the phrenic nerve may result in slow regeneration with restoration of function. The incidence of ice slush-induced phrenic nerve dysfunction has been reported between 27% and 73%.[9,10] Overall, the incidence of diaphragmatic paralysis after cardiac surgery is 0.3% to 12.8%.[11] Another etiology is related to blood supply of the phrenic nerve: 70% of the blood supply to the phrenic nerve comes from the IMA, with the nerve and artery in closer proximity on the right side. High cephalad dissection of the right IMA increases the risk of phrenic nerve injury. In a retrospective analysis, the incidence of right-sided diaphragm paralysis after right internal mammary harvest was found to be 4%.[12] When comparing right and left phrenic nerve injuries, right-sided injury is more likely to result in noticeable respiratory dysfunction.[13] The STOP AF trial reported 11.2% of patients developed phrenic nerve palsy after cryoablation for atrial fibrillation, with 86% resolving at 12 months.[14] In a study of postsurgical diaphragm paralysis, there was a 32% incidence of unilateral paralysis in patients when topical ice or hypothermia was used, though nearly all showed eventual recovery with conservative management at 2 years.[15] Unless the patient has severe associated respiratory dysfunction in the postoperative setting, surgical repair should be deferred to an outpatient setting, with reevaluation over time to monitor recovery of diaphragm function.

Complete transection or direct injury to the phrenic nerve has a low change of spontaneous recovery. Mechanisms of injury include surgery on the chest or neck, crushing forces, traction injury, nerve transection, or thermal injury. In the neck, phrenic nerve injury has been reported after scalenectomy for thoracic outlet syndrome, radical neck dissection, and blunt trauma to the neck. Abdominal surgery also carries risk; right hemidiaphragm paralysis has been reported in up to 79% of patients secondary to injury during cross clamping of the suprahepatic vena cava in orthotopic liver transplants. If there is evidence of

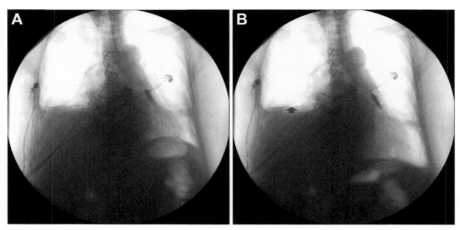

Fig. 3. Fluoroscopy demonstrating abnormal sniff test with paradoxic motion of the right diaphragm. (*A*) The right hemidiaphragm is elevated at rest. (*B*) During inspiration, the left diaphragm has normal downward excursion (*blue arrow*), whereas the right diaphragm has paradoxic elevation (*purple arrow*).

traumatic injury or transection of the phrenic nerve, spontaneous recovery of diaphragm function will not occur. Some patients with nerve injury are potential candidates for nerve transfer[16] or phrenic nerve pacing,[17] both of which are outside the scope of this article.

INDICATIONS FOR SURGERY IN DIAPHRAGM PARALYSIS AND EVENTRATION

Surgical plication is the treatment of choice for both symptomatic eventration and diaphragm paralysis. First described in the early twentieth century by Wood and Morrison[18], the goal of diaphragm plication is to immobilize the diaphragm into a lower and flatter position to reduce paradoxic movement allowing for functional recovery with adequate muscle reserve.[18] Initially, diaphragm plication was performed via a thoracotomy or a laparotomy. Today, minimally invasive options such as video-assisted thoracoscopic surgery (VATS) and robotic surgery have become the preferred approach.

Plication is indicated in patients with diaphragm elevation and persistent or limiting symptoms. Common indications for intervention in adults include severe dyspnea, orthopnea, or severe decline in PFT or exercise tolerance. In a study by Deng and colleagues, patients with transection of the right phrenic nerve who underwent immediate diaphragmatic plication had forced vital capacities of 0.90 L, compared with 0.79 L for those diagnosed with phrenic nerve dysfunction who had no treatment.[12] If diaphragm elevation is long-standing and the patient is asymptomatic then surgical intervention may also be indicated, though there are no clear guidelines on which

patients may benefit most. Of note, morbid obesity is a relative contraindication to surgery, as the elevated intra-abdominal pressure can result in increased failure of the surgical plication.

DIAPHRAGM PLICATION

The goal of plication is to reduce paradoxic excursion during inspiration. The procedure improves symptoms by increasing both inspiratory and expiratory lung volumes as lowering the cupola allows for better re-expansion of the adjacent lung. A successful plication will provide satisfactory tension to an abnormally flask-shaped dome while simultaneously lowering it. Flattening the diaphragm also improves the actions of the intercostal and accessory muscles.

Plication can be approached via thoracotomy, laparotomy, or more contemporarily through a minimally invasive approach. A laparoscopic approach from the abdomen is useful if there is infradiaphragmatic involvement or gastric volvulus involved. In the absence of bilateral disease or gastric involvement, an intrathoracic approach is preferred. Repair is most often performed via plication using sutures. Although the use of endostaplers for diaphragm plication or resection of the diaphragm with primary repair have been described, this is not the authors preferred approach due to the potential risk of dehiscence of the staple or suture line, which would result in a large diaphragmatic hernia.

Thoracotomy

An open thoracotomy with suture plication was previously the standard of care for symptomatic eventration or paralysis. Using single-lung ventilation, the sixth, seventh, or eighth interspace posterolateral thoracotomy is created, depending on the height of the dysfunctional diaphragm. The diaphragm can be plicated from medial to lateral until the surface is taut and flat. A variety of fixation sutures can be used, such as interrupted or running mattress sutures, interrupted U stitches, or running sutures to fold the diaphragm on itself.[19] All sutures should be heavy, nonabsorbable suture, with or without pledgets to buttress the repair. Multiple overlapping layers are often performed to decrease the likelihood of dehiscence and to get an adequate flattening of the diaphragm with an appropriate amount of tension.

Before chest closure, it is imperative to re-inflate the lung under direct visualization. For some patients with prior surgery or trauma, there may be intrathoracic adhesions that restrict the lung from fully inflating. If adhesions are present, a thorough adhesiolysis is necessary for the lung to fill the thoracic cavity and allow the patient to benefit from the plication.

Transabdominal Approach

Abdominal approaches to diaphragm plication may be performed laparoscopically or open. The position of the liver makes transabdominal diaphragm plication more difficult on the right compared with the left, though this approach has been described for both hemidiaphragms. An open transabdominal plication is generally performed via midline laparotomy, though some have described a transverse laparotomy as well. After abdominal entry, the diaphragm is grasped with two Babcock forceps and drawn downward to flatten the diaphragm. A pleat is created with the mattress sutures going from the base and folding to the anterior circumference of the diaphragm.

Laparoscopic and robotic diaphragm plication is now more common than an open transabdominal approach. The patient is placed in a 30° reverse Trendelenburg position with the surgeon standing between the legs and one assistant on either side. A 30° scope is introduced through a paraumbilical incision. Three additional working ports are placed in a semicircle in the right or left middle and upper abdomen. The left hepatic lobe is mobilized along the left triangular ligament, and three retention stitches are placed transcutaneously. By application of extracorporeal traction, the diaphragm dome is able to be reduced and an intra-abdominal fold is created. Generally, 12 to 15 nonabsorbable U-stitches are placed along the

fold. These can be tied intracorporeally or extracorporeally and then cinched down with a knot pusher.[19] There is a small risk of splenic or liver injury using this approach. A potential drawback to the transabdominal minimally invasive approach is the insufflation required for visualization which pushes the diaphragm cephalad. To counter this, a small thoracoscopic port with thoracic insufflation may be used to deflect the diaphragm downward.[20] A small hole can be made in the diaphragm as well to equalize the pressure between the chest and abdomen.[21] Multiple layers of imbricating sutures are performed from medial to lateral, starting at the posterior aspect of the diaphragm. Again, heavy nonabsorbable suture is used for the repair. At the end of the procedure, if a thoracic trocar was used, a chest tube is placed through the thoracoscopic trocar site.[20]

Advantages to the transabdominal approach are the ability to plicate both hemidiaphragms if there is bilateral paralysis as well as avoiding single-lung ventilation. However, if there are adhesions of the lung, these cannot be taken down from this approach. There is also decreased visualization of the right hemidiaphragm and potential inadvertent injury to the lung.

Video-Assisted Thoracoscopic Surgery

A VATS approach is commonly used for diaphragm plication, with variations including a three-port approach or uniportal approach. In both, the patient is placed in a lateral decubitus position, and single-lung ventilation is used.

The most commonly used port configuration placed two ports in the eighth intercostal space and one in the fifth intercostal space. Insufflation can be used to help flatten the diaphragm and aid in the plication. A variety of techniques have been described, each effectively achieving lowering of the diaphragm. Some surgeons perform rows of interrupted sutures from the cardiophrenic angle to the lateral chest wall, until the diaphragm is flattened.[22] Others use the Endostitch device to place multiple, pledgeted U stitches (generally 8–15) to plicate the diaphragm.[23]

Another technique described by Demos and colleagues includes a 5 cm working incision at the level of the ideal position of the dome of the diaphragm post-plication (often the eighth or ninth interspace), a second port in the fifth intercostal space in the anterior axillary line, and another port 2 interspaces above the working port and 3 to 4 cm posteriorly.[24] Insufflation is not used, due to the large size of the working port, and the diaphragm is pushed down with thoracoscopic

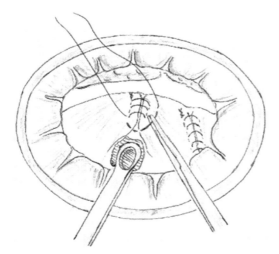

Fig. 4. Uniportal video-assisted thoracoscopic surgery view with an Alexis wound retractor and running horizontal mattress suture.

instruments. A #1 polypropylene suture is run in horizontal mattress style beginning posterolaterally and running anteromedially, plicating a width of diaphragm approximately 5 cm. Once the anteromedial extent is reached, the suture is then reversed and two new folds of diaphragm are captured, extending out another few centimeters on either side depending on how much additional lowering the diaphragm requires to achieve an ideal result.[24]

A uniportal approach is performed through a 4-cm incision in the ninth interspace, midaxillary line, and a small wound retractor is placed. A thoracoscope is inserted through this incision to help with visualization. The diaphragm is pushed downward, and a running horizontal mattress is performed from medial to lateral with heavy suture (#2 polyester or #1 polypropylene are preferred sutures). Two more layers of running horizontal mattress sutures are performed for three total layers of plication. Although **Fig. 4** shows the suture lines in parallel, we often perform our plication suture over one another for overlapping layers. Each layer is adjusted to ultimately achieve the right position and tension on the diaphragm. Postoperative CXR demonstrates significant downward displacement of the diaphragm (**Fig. 5**A, B). Similar to thoracotomy, it is essential to ensure the lung inflates completely at the end of the case to fill the thoracic cavity. If needed, adhesiolysis should be performed.

Robotic-Assisted Thoracic Surgery

Robotic-assisted thoracic surgery is now a very common approach for diaphragm plication. The patient is placed in a lateral decubitus semi-flexed position and single-lung ventilation is used. A variety of port placements have been described.[25–27] Our preferred port placement is shown in **Fig. 6**; an 8 mm port is placed in the fifth or sixth intercostal space anterior to the scapular tip, and insufflation is used. Two more 8 mm ports are placed anteriorly and one posteriorly in the same interspace. An assist port is placed as inferiorly as possible. The robot is turned 180° then docked.

The most common method for robotic diaphragm plication is an "accordion" plication. The redundant diaphragm is pulled in a radial direction and pleats are created using full-thickness horizontal mattress sutures in the anteromedial to

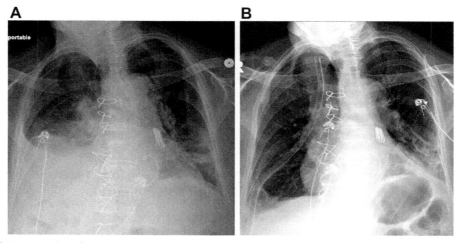

Fig. 5. (*A*) Preoperative chest radiography with elevated right hemidiaphragm. (*B*) Postoperative chest radiography after uniportal right diaphragm plication.

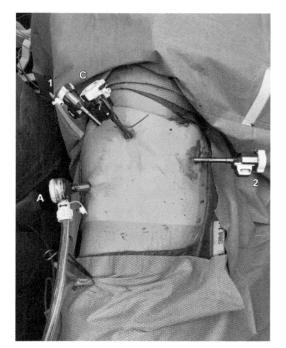

Fig. 6. Robotic port placement for diaphragm plication. The camera port is labeled C, the assist port is labeled A, and ports 1 and 2 label the right and left hands, respectively.

posteromedial direction while avoiding phrenic nerve branches. As shown in **Fig. 7**A, the sutures are buttressed with pledgets and a heavy nonabsorbable suture, such as #2 polyester is used. Although we previously performed intracorporeal knots, we now use a core-knot to create the maximum flattening of the diaphragm with appropriate tension. Roughly 8 to 12 sutures are needed to complete the plication (**Fig. 7**B). At the end of the procedure, a chest tube is placed and the lung should be inflated under direct visualization. Adhesiolysis should be performed if necessary.

POSTOPERATIVE MANAGEMENT

A chest tube is placed in all patients who undergo a diaphragm plication. The chest tube can frequently be removed on postoperative day (POD) 1, with standard criteria for chest tube removal such as no air leak and minimal fluid output. Many patients are discharged after VATS or robotic diaphragm plication on POD 1. For patients who undergo an open repair via thoracotomy, pain management is often the rate limiting step with the need for epidural or intercostal nerve cryoablation, requiring a longer length of stay.

Owing to the possibility of increased abdominal pressure causing the diaphragm plication sutures to tear, postoperative recovery includes the avoidance of heavy lifting and strenuous core exercises. A good bowel regimen is important to prevent constipation, which can result in unnecessary tension on the repair in the postoperative setting.

Patients should return to the clinic for a postoperative CXR to assess the plication as well as for postoperative pleural effusion. Patients who undergo diaphragm plication may develop a postoperative effusion secondary to the increase in intrathoracic space. For small effusions, conservative management is often effective. However, patients who develop postoperative dyspnea secondary to an effusion may require thoracentesis.

OUTCOMES

Studies of diaphragm plication have shown that it is a safe and effective procedure, with improvement in PFTs and dyspnea levels.[28–30] Data have demonstrated the safety and efficacy of VATS[24] and robotic plication,[25] with decreased length of stay compared with thoracotomy. Studies have shown that in cases of known phrenic nerve transection, a diaphragm plication during the index operation can prevent pulmonary complications and preserve lung function.[12]

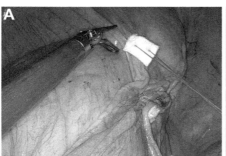
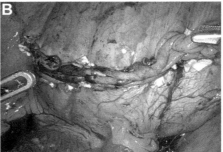

Fig. 7. Robotic accordion diaphragm plication. (*A*) the initial suture is placed with multiple bites of diaphragm with pledgets to buttress both ends of the stitch. (*B*) The final plication with multiple pledgeted stitches showing the plicated diaphragm.

Although diaphragm plication is well described with defined criteria for repair in the pediatric population, the adult population lacks this clarity and timing and need for intervention remain debated. There is greater consensus for symptomatic adult patients, but further studies are needed to define the benefits of early surgery in the asymptomatic adult patient with phrenic nerve paralysis or incidentally found large eventration. The development of minimally invasive techniques for diaphragm plication have shortened recovery time and diminished the morbidity associated with this procedure potentially expanding the pool of operative candidates.

CLINICS CARE POINTS

- Eventration refers to elevation of one or both hemidiaphragms due to decreased muscle fibers. It may present as a congenital defect or be acquired.
- Diaphragm paralysis is an acquired condition resulting in elevation of one or both hemidiaphragms due to disruption or disease of the phrenic.
- Diaphragm elevation is often an incidental finding on chest radiographs.
- The "Sniff test" is a fluoroscopic examination that can help determine whether there is phrenic nerve involvement in cases of diaphragm elevation found on imaging.
- Both direct and indirect iatrogenic phrenic nerve injuries may be difficult to appreciate at the time of cardiothoracic surgery. Awareness of the possibility of injury and knowledge of the relevant anatomy is the best defense against accidental injury. Some phrenic nerve injuries may heal spontaneously.
- In adults, plication is indicated in patients with diaphragm elevation and persistent symptoms.
- The goal of plication is to reduce paradoxic excursion during inspiration. The procedure improves symptoms by increasing both inspiratory and expiratory lung volumes.
- A successful plication will provide satisfactory tension while flattening the diaphragm.
- Plication can be approached open or minimally invasively via the chest or abdomen.
- In adult patients, diaphragm plication in non-ventilator-dependent patients carries a relatively low operative risk and generally results in improved functionality and improvement in symptoms.

- Indications and timing for diaphragm plication are still debated in the adult population for asymptomatic patients.

DISCLOSURE

The authors have no relevant financial disclosures.

REFERENCES

1. Shields TW. Embryology and anatomy of the diaphragm. In: Locicero J, Feins RH, Colson YL, et al, editors. Shield's general thoracic surgery. 8th edition. Philadelphia: Wolters Kluwer; 2019. p. 659–63.
2. Dubé BP, Dres M. Diaphragm dysfunction: diagnostic approaches and management strategies. J Clin Med 2016;5(12):113.
3. Schumpelick V, Steinau G, Schluper I, et al. Surgical embryology and anatomy of the diaphragm with surgical applications. Surg Clin North Am 2000;80(1):213–39.
4. Piehler JM, Pairolero PC, Gracey DR, et al. Unexplained diaphragmatic paralysis: a harbinger of malignant disease? J Thorac Cardiovasc Surg 1982;84(6):861–4.
5. Suwatanapongched T, Gierada DS, Slone RM, et al. Variation in diaphragm position and shape in adults with normal pulmonary function. Chest 2003;123(6):2019–27.
6. Willaert W, Kessler R, Deneffe G. Surgical options for complete resectable lung cancer invading the phrenic nerve. Acta Chir Belg 2004;104(4):451–3.
7. Lisboa C, Pare PD, Pertuze J, et al. Inspiratory muscle function in unilateral diaphragmatic paralysis. Am Rev Respir Dis 1986;134:488–92.
8. Laroche CM, Carroll N, Moxham J, et al. Clinical significance of severe isolated diaphragm weakness. Am Rev Respir Dis 1988;138:862–6.
9. Dimopoulou I, Daganou M, Dafni U, et al. Phrenic nerve dysfunction after cardiac operations: electrophysiologic evaluation of risk factors. Chest 1998;113(1):8–14.
10. Rousou JA, Parker T, Engelman RM, et al. Phrenic nerve paresis associated with the use of iced slush and the cooling jacket for topical hypothermia. J Thorac Cardiovasc Surg 1985;89(6):921–5.
11. Joho-Arreola AL, Bauersfeld U, Stauffer UG, et al. Incidence and treatment of diaphragmatic paralysis after cardiac surgery in children. Eur J Cardio Thorac Surg 2005;27(1):53–7.
12. Deng Y, Byth K, Paterson HS. Phrenic nerve injury associated with high free right internal mammary artery harvesting. Ann Thorac Surg 2003;76(2):459–63.
13. Lai DT, Paterson HS. Mini-thoracotomy for diaphragmatic plication with thoracoscopic assistance. Ann Thorac Surg 1999;68(6):2364–5.

14. Packer DL, Kowal RC, Wheelan KR, et al. Cryoballoon ablation of pulmonary veins for paroxysmal atrial fibrillation: first results of the North American Arctic Front (STOP AF) pivotal trial. J Am Coll Cardiol 2013;61(16):1713–23.

15. Efthimiou J, Butler J, Woodham C, et al. Diaphragm paralysis following cardiac surgery: role of phrenic nerve cold injury. Ann Thorac Surg 1991;52(4): 1005–8.

16. Moore AM, Wagner IJ, Fox IK. Principles of nerve repair in complex wounds of the upper extremity. Semin Plast Surg 2015;29(1):40–7.

17. Chalidapong P, Sananpanich K, Kraisarin J, et al. Pulmonary and biceps function after intercostal and phrenic nerve transfer for brachial plexus injuries. J Hand Surg Br 2004;29(1):8–11.

18. Wood HG. Eventration of the diaphragm. Surg Gynecol Obstet 1916;23:344.

19. Huttl TP, Wichmann MW, Reichart B, et al. Laparoscopic diaphragmatic plication: long-term results of a novel surgical technique for postoperative phrenic nerve palsy. Surg Endosc 2004;18:547–51.

20. Onders RP. Physiology of the diaphragm and surgical approaches to the paralyzed diaphragm. In: Locicero J, Feins RH, Colson YL, et al, editors. Shield's general thoracic surgery. 8th edition. Philadelphia: Wolters Kluwer; 2019. p. 664–72.

21. Roy SB, Haworth C, Ipsen T, et al. Transabdominal robot-assisted diaphragmatic plication: a 3.5 year experience. Eur J Cardio Thorac Surg 2018;53(1): 247–53.

22. Vieira A, Ugalde P. Available at:. In: CTSNet, editor. VATS technique for diaphragm plication. 2019 https:// www.ctsnet.org/article/vats-technique-diaphragmatic-plication. [Accessed 9 August 2023]; 2019.

23. Dunning J. Thoracoscopic diaphragm plication. Interact Cardiovasc Thorac Surg 2015;20(5): 689–90.

24. Demos DS, Berry MF, Backhus LM, et al. Video-assisted thoracoscopic diaphragm plication using a running suture technique is durable and effective. J Thorac Cardiovasc Surg 2017;153(5):1182–8.

25. Schumacher L, Zhao D. Outcomes and technique of robotic diaphragm plication. J Thorac Dis 2021; 13(10):6113–5.

26. Asaf BB, Gopinath SK, Kumar A, et al. Robotic diaphragm plication for eventration: a retrospective analysis of efficacy, safety, and feasibility. Asian J Endosc Surg 2021;14(1):70–6.

27. Gilbert A, Wei B. Diaphragmatic plication: current evidence and techniques in the management of the elevated hemidiaphragm. Video-assist Thorac Surg 2023;8:16.

28. Celik S, Celik M, Aydemir B, et al. Long-term results of diaphragmatic plication in adults with unilateral diaphragm paralysis. J Cardiothorac Surg 2010;5: 111.

29. Versteegh MIM, Braun J, Voigt PG, et al. Diaphragm plication in adult patients with diaphragm paralysis leads to long-term improvement of pulmonary function and level of dyspnea. Eur J Cardio Thorac Surg 2007;32(3):449–56.

30. Simanksy DA, Paley M, Yellin A. Diaphragm plication following phrenic nerve injury: a comparison of paediatric and adult patients. Thorax 2002;57:613–6.

Management of Diaphragm Tumors

Marta Engelking, MD[a],*, Madhuri Rao, MD[b]

KEYWORDS

- Diaphragm tumors • Cyst • Lipoma • Rhabdomyosarcoma • Leiomyosarcoma • Endometriosis
- Diaphragm reconstruction

KEY POINTS

- Tumors of the diaphragm are quite rare, with secondary tumors being more common than primary tumors, whether benign or malignant.
- Tumors of the diaphragm are often incidental findings, but if symptomatic or there is concern for malignancy, complete resection is preferred.
- Surgical resection may require partial or complete resection of the diaphragm, focusing on a tension-free primary repair versus reconstruction, with the use of autologous tissue or mesh.

INTRODUCTION

Tumors of the diaphragm are the rarest tumor of the intrathoracic cavity. Primary tumors, whether benign or malignant, have about the same occurrence rate. The most common benign primary tumors are diaphragmatic cyst and lipomas, and the most common malignant primary tumors are rhabdomyosarcoma and fibromyosarcoma.[1,2] Weksler and Ginsberg's review of the literature evaluated cases in 106 patients, revealing an equal distribution between males and females, representation of all age groups from 18 months to 76 years, and equally involved right and left hemidiaphragms.[1]

Secondary tumors of the diaphragm are far more common involving both malignant and benign etiologies—endometriosis accounting for the majority of benign cases. Spread may occur via direct extension from thoracic and abdominal tumors into the diaphragm or seeding of the pleural or peritoneal space.

Publications detailing diaphragmatic tumors date back to 1955, but due to their rarity, most of the publications are case reports and case series that have cumulatively contributed to about 200 total cases.[1,3–5]

Most of the diaphragmatic tumors are found incidentally on chest imaging—historically chest x-ray and more contemporarily on computed tomography (CT) scans. Symptoms are nonspecific and generally present when a tumor has reached a sufficient size to impact surrounding structures and manifest. Most commonly these manifest with chest pain, abdominal pain, and cough.[1] CT imaging is helpful to delineate the mass and its characteristics, to help aid in diagnosis, and plan therapy. In most cases, a biopsy is required to assist with diagnosis and guide care. This article outlines the details of these rare tumors to provide a basic understanding of the diagnosis and management.

PRIMARY TUMORS OF THE DIAPHRAGM

Benign Primary Tumors

Lipomatous tumors

Lipomas and cysts are the most common benign primary tumors reported, though lipomas are now thought to be more common than cystic lesions.

Typically, lipomas are asymptomatic unless large enough to cause compression of adjacent

[a] Department of General Surgery, Division of Thoracic & Foregut Surgery, University of Minnesota, 420 Delaware Street Southeast, MMC 207, Minneapolis, MN 55455, USA; [b] Division of Thoracic and Foregut Surgery, University of Minnesota, 420 Delaware Street Southeast, MMC 207, Minneapolis, MN 55455, USA
* Corresponding author. Division of Thoracic & Foregut Surgery, University of Minnesota, 420 Delaware Street Southeast, MMC 207, Minneapolis, MN 55455.
E-mail address: engel897@umn.edu

Thorac Surg Clin 34 (2024) 189–195
https://doi.org/10.1016/j.thorsurg.2024.01.009
1547-4127/24/© 2024 Elsevier Inc. All rights reserved.

structures or pain. The first documented dia-phragm lipoma dates back to 1886.[6-12] These tu-mors are soft, circumscribed, and encapsulated fatty tumors. CT classically reveals a homogenous lesion filled with Hounsfield units consistent with adipose tissue, which is diagnostic. Concerning features would include heterogeneity and enhancing solid components, which should prompt resection, even if not symptomatic, given the risk for malignancy over time.[13,14]

Cystic tumors

There are two primary types of diaphragmatic cysts: mesothelial and bronchogenic. Although cysts are most often found incidentally, symptoms increase with growth of the cyst and may include upper abdominal pain, cough, or shortness of breath. Isolated case reports describe most commonly symptoms arising once the cyst has become large enough to compress surrounding structures.[6-8]

Mesothelial cysts are congenital cysts arising from coelomic remnants of the adrenal, ovary, falciform ligament, spleen, mesentery, and rarely the diaphragm. These may be diagnosed in chil-dren or adults. Ultrasound can assist with diag-nosis and reveals a thin-walled cystic structure. CT shows a homogenous, nonenhancing, well-defined cyst, with water density. Diagnosis is typi-cally made based on these imaging findings. There is some evidence to suggest mesothelial cysts will regress or resolve completely with time, though this is only described with children. Typical ther-apy options include percutaneous aspiration, sclerotherapy, or surgical resection.[6-8]

Bronchogenic cysts are another developmental anomaly arising from the foregut, usually within the mediastinum or lung parenchyma, resulting in aberrant buds from the tracheobronchial tree. Im-aging has shown a large bulging mass over the diaphragm with a hypoechoic lesion on CT or MRI, difficult to distinguish between other types of cysts. Most commonly these lesions have been resected via laparoscopy or video-assisted thoracoscopic surgery (VATS), though enucleation has also been described.[9-11]

Other benign primary tumors

Less commonly described are other primary benign tumors including hydatid cyst from *Echino-coccus granulosus*, chondroma, schwannoma, hemangioma, neurofibroma, angiofibroma, endo-thelioma, and leiomyoma. Surgical resection was performed in nearly all cases, as reports are too rare to determine safety of conservative manage-ment and risk of malignancy.[15-17]

Malignant Primary Tumors

Rhabdomyosarcoma

Rhabdomyosarcoma and leiomyosarcoma are two more commonly documented malignant pri-mary diaphragmatic tumors. Rhabdomyosarcoma is a malignant tumor arising from embryonic mesenchymal cells, which can differentiate into skeletal muscle cells. There are four histologic classifications: pleomorphic, alveolar, botryoid, and embryonal. These are typically found in chil-dren, most commonly in the head/neck, urogenital tract and extremities, but in rare case reports arise from the diaphragm.[18] Most patients are asymp-tomatic or present with vague complaints of chest pain, cough, or dyspnea. CT imaging shows a het-erogeneous, enhancing mass, and diagnosis can be made on histology with imaging-guided biopsy. Treatment routinely involves chemotherapy and resection, with a questionable benefit from radia-tion therapy.[19]

Leiomyosarcoma

Leiomyosarcoma is a malignant neoplasm of smooth muscle and is one of the most common subtypes of soft tissue sarcoma. Most commonly this arises from the uterus, with origin from the diaphragm contributing a small number of cases.[20] CT imaging shows a heterogeneous mass of low density, and MRI can help differen-tiate these features, with a low signal on T1 and iso-intensity on T2. For localized, resectable dis-ease, surgery is the mainstay of therapy.[20-23] Unresectable tumors, and those who develop recurrence or metastatic disease, have multiple lines of chemotherapy (first line and beyond first line) options, as well as immunotherapy and new targeted therapies.[24]

Other primary malignant tumors

Other rare primary malignancies have been re-ported, including malignant schwannoma,[16] lipo-sarcoma,[13,14] yolk sac tumor,[1,25] osteosarcoma,[26] and other forms of sarcoma including Ewing sar-coma[27] and synovial sarcoma.[28-44] Routinely, complete resection has been performed for these rare tumors (**Figs. 1–3**).

BENIGN SECONDARY TUMORS
Endometriosis

Endometriosis is described as the most common benign metastatic disease found on the dia-phragm. Endometriosis is ectopic growth of endo-metrial stromal and glandular tissue, which is found outside the uterine cavity, and is theorized to occur secondary to retrograde menstruation. Lesions are most commonly found within the

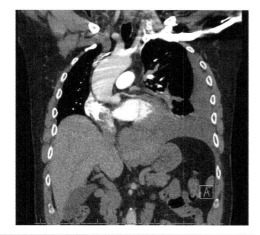

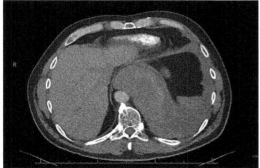

Fig. 1. A 7.3 × 5.0 cm mass involving the left diaphragmatic crus, left lung, and left pleura, in a patient presenting with dyspnea and syncope. Biopsy showed synovial sarcoma.

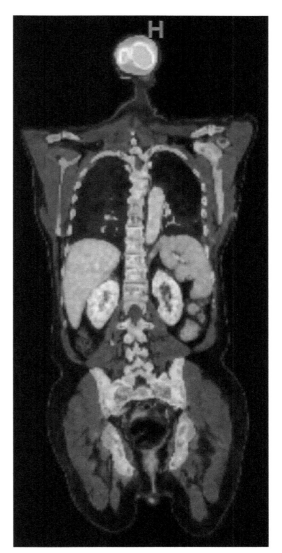

Fig.   2. PET-CT   performed   post-chemotherapy treatment.

pelvis but may be found on the peritoneal and in some cases pleural side of the diaphragm. Women often present with upper abdominal pain, shoulder pain, chest pain, or shortness of breath. Occasionally, asymptomatic cases are identified. Symptoms are often cyclical, developing within 72 hours of menstruation, and can be complicated by catamenial pneumothorax, hemothorax, or hemoptysis.[28–31] CT imaging may identify a mass, but this is often indeterminate. MRI is the best for diagnosis by appearance of hemorrhage and surrounding low-intensity rings. It is unclear why, but 70% to 80% of cases have favored the right diaphragm.

The first-line treatment is medical therapy with hormone suppression, which is often initiated without histologic diagnosis. If complicated disease including pneumothorax or hemothorax is involved, this must be addressed first with chest tube drainage, followed by a plan for decreasing the risk of recurrence, including mechanical or chemical pleurodesis.[26] Once the acute phase has resolved, long-term management includes ongoing medical therapy, with ablation and/or resection reserved for progress of disease or failure of medical therapy.[30–32] Surgical management can therefore include resection of the involved diaphragm, fenestration with closure of the diaphragm, or pleurodesis, all while continuing medical therapy to avoid the necessity of a total abdominal hysterectomy.[29,32,33]

Local Malignant Secondary Tumors

Malignancies may arise on either side of the diaphragm and invade into the structure. This can include intrathoracic malignancies such as mesothelioma, esophageal cancer, or lung cancer, as well as intra-abdominal malignancies including

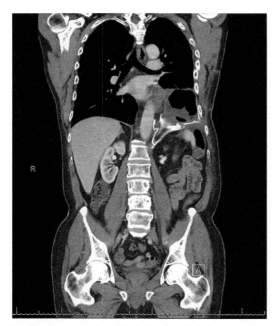

Fig. 3. Postoperative CT following left lower lobectomy with en bloc resection of partial left hemidiaphragm with mesh reconstruction.

hepatic, renal, retroperitoneal, and other gastrointestinal (GI) primaries. Fortunately, these findings do not necessarily preclude resection of the primary disease, as en bloc resection can often be performed with repair of the diaphragm.[2]

The most common local malignancy involving the diaphragm is lung cancer. Patients with advanced lung cancer may develop pleural involvement and/or pleural effusion, with invasion of the diaphragm occurring in less than 0.5% of patients.[34–36] These tumors are classified as T4, but the presence of diaphragm involvement does not change the management plan. Studies evaluating patients with advanced lung cancer in whom there is localized in invasion without wide spread disease, found that with complete en bloc resection 5-year survival rates range from 20 to 30 months, with local recurrence up to 40% and distant recurrence up to 79%.[34–37] Unfortunately, the most common presentation of advanced lung disease with diaphragm involvement has more advanced, widespread disease, and therefore, resection is typically not an option in those cases.

Although malignant mesothelioma is rare, at the time of presentation the extent of disease commonly includes the visceral and parietal pleural as well as diaphragm. Partial or complete resection of the diaphragm is often required to obtain appropriate negative margins.

Esophageal cancer near the gastroesophageal (GE) junction can directly invade the diaphragm at the crus, as well as gastric cancer of the cardia or GI stromal tumor. If the underlying malignancy is deemed resectable, the disease portion of diaphragm is resected en bloc, and depending the extent of resection, may or may not require hiatal reconstruction.[39]

Malignant Metastatic Tumors

Malignancies rarely metastasize to the diaphragm, but there are a few that have been described. Endometrial cancer is probably the furthest primary cancer which has been found to spread to the diaphragm, as evidence suggests it is more common for a thoracic primary to metastasize here. "Drop metastases" refers to tumors that form within the pleural space and directly shed tumor cells within the cavity, leading to metastatic disease. Thymomas have been reported to spread in this manner, often in cases of recurrence. A thymoma is an epithelial tumor within the anterior mediastinum, with many subtypes. Although seen on CT imaging, diagnosis is most reliable with image-guided biopsy or thoracoscopy. Drop metastases are generally thought to represent advanced disease but can be resected to provide local control and prolonged disease-free survival.[2,40,41]

Management

Observation can be a safe management strategy for tumors which are well defined on imaging and do not show characteristics concerning for malignant pathology. As previously mentioned, this includes straight forward lipomas and benign cysts. Endometriosis is another benign process which is typically managed medically, but may eventually require surgical intervention.

Percutaneous biopsy can be a helpful diagnostic tool to determine if resection should be performed. This can also be helpful to facilitate clear margins during surgery. However, depending on the location of the tumor, it may not be accessible or feasible to perform safely, therefore VATS or diagnostic laparoscopy may be indicated for further evaluation. In addition, depending on the tumor, biopsy may not be sufficient for diagnosis, and sensitivity may be low; therefore, if suspicion for malignancy is high, resection would be indicated.

In some individual cases, induction chemotherapy may be indicated. This is relatively well documented in case studies of rare types of sarcoma. However, more recently, this has been reserved for metastatic or particularly high-risk cases. Unfortunately, as with many of these tumors, they are so rare, no definitive recommendations exist for multimodal treatment regimens; however, with the expansion of treatment options including immunotherapy and targeted therapies, this will continue to evolve.[24,45–51]

Complete resection is the primary goal of surgical management of diaphragm tumors. Small tumors may undergo a partial resection, but removal of the hemidiaphragm may be required depending on the diagnosis and the extent of tumor involvement. A detailed understanding of anatomy is essential to a safe resection. The diaphragm is the major involuntary muscle of respiration and separates the abdominal and thoracic cavities. The left and right phrenic nerves originate at C3–5 and run along the mediastinum to innervate the diaphragm. Injury to these nerves results in diaphragm paralysis. The blood supply includes the phrenic artery and vein, as well as the intercostals. The right and left sides then form the diaphragmatic crus, through which the aorta runs posterior along the left, the inferior vena cava (IVC) on the right, and anteriorly the esophagus (**Fig. 4**).[45]

Resection with primary closure of the diaphragm is possible in cases in which the muscle is brought together without tension. For primary repair, the authors recommend using nonabsorbable interrupted sutures with pledgets. Primary repair comes with the risk of diaphragmatic hernia, specifically for those who undergo concomitant peritonectomy and either neoadjuvant or adjuvant chemotherapy due to concern for wound healing.[52] However, this is not well studied in the literature overall (**Figs. 5** and **6**).

In any case where there is concern for tension of the tissues, or with large defects or complete resection of the hemidiaphragm, reconstruction

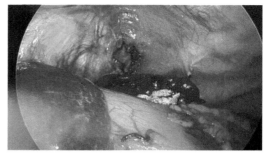
Fig. 5. Laparoscopic partial diaphragm resection.

should be performed. There are options of synthetic or autologous tissue reconstructions. Mesh reconstruction was previously performed routinely with Marlex, which is a heavy polypropylene mesh. More recently, flexible polytetrafluoroethylene mesh is preferred. The mesh is measured in two dimensions and cut to fit the defect. In cases of patch repair of a partial resection, the mesh is secured with nonabsorbable suture to the remaining diaphragm edges or secured around ribs to the chest wall. For complete resections, it is useful to leave a rim of diaphragm medially to which the mesh can be anchored using interrupted or running suture. The mesh is secured along the ribs anteriorly, laterally, and posteriorly. This should be along the seventh rib anteriorly and the tenth rib posteriorly, to follow the natural course of the diaphragm, ensuring a watertight closure. This closure is more critical on the left hemidiaphragm, given the potential herniation of the contents of the abdominal cavity, without the protective presence of the liver.[38,43,47] Muscle flaps are a well-documented autologous reconstruction option. A pedicled muscle flap was first described by Rosenkratz using the latissimus dorsi muscle.[46] This has since expanded to other options, including the serratus anterior, rectus abdominis, external oblique, and transversus abdominis, primarily described in the pediatric population.[49]

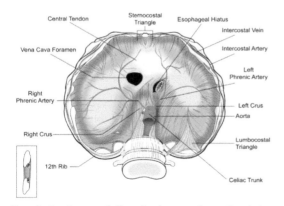
Fig. 4. Anatomy of the diaphragm from the intra-abdominal space. (*From* Finley DJ, Abu-Rustum NR, Chi DS et al. Reconstructive techniques after diaphragm resection. Thorac Surg Clin 2009;19(4):175-180.)

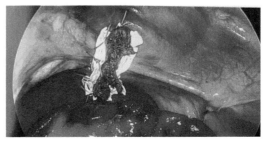
Fig. 6. Complete laparoscopic diaphragm repair with interrupted reinforced sutures.

SUMMARY

Diaphragm tumors are the rarest tumor of the thorax, with secondary tumors being more common than primary. The most common benign primary tumors include lipomas and cysts, and malignant primary tumors include rhabdomyosarcoma and leiomyosarcoma. Endometriosis is the most common benign secondary tumor, followed by malignant tumors with localized spread of disease from lung cancer, mesothelioma, the GE junction, and the mediastinum. In addition, widely metastatic disease from ovarian or endometrial cancers has been described. Documentation of these tumors is mostly through case reports. Management can be conservative in a diagnostically certain benign processes like a lipoma or simple cyst. If imaging is inconclusive, percutaneous biopsy or diagnostic VATS or laparoscopy may be an additional diagnostic tool. With any concerning radiographic or biopsy findings, resection is recommended. With partial resection, the diaphragm can often be repaired primarily, though any large defect or tension would indicate the need for mesh or an autologous reconstruction.

CLINICS CARE POINTS

- Diaphragm tumors are rare and mostly described through case reports, so there is little detail describing a consensus in the appropriate management of these rare cases.

- Typically confirmed benign diseases such as small lipomas and cysts are managed conservatively.

- Most of other tumors are managed with resection, with the exception of widespread metastatic cancers and endometriosis.

- Partial diaphragm resection can be repaired primarily if able to achieve a tension-free closure.

- Surgeons should have a low threshold for placement of mesh or consideration of reconstruction to ensure appropriate healing and function of the diaphragm.

DISCLOSURE

The authors have nothing to disclose.

REFERENCES

1. Weksler B, Ginsberg RJ. Tumors of the diaphragm. Chest Surg Clin 1998;8(2):441–7.

2. Kim MP, Hofstetter WL. Tumors of the diaphragm. Thorac Surg Clin 2009;19(4):521–9.

3. Weiner MF, Chou WH. Primary tumor of the diaphragm. Arch Surg 1965;90:143–52.

4. Olafsson C, Rausing A, Holen O. Primary tumors of the diaphragm. Chest 1970;59. 598-570.

5. Mordant P, Le Pimpec-Barthes F, Gangi A, et al. Tumours of the diaphragm. In: Juzdal J, editor. ESTS Textbook of thoracic surgery. Cracow (Poland): Medycyna Praktyczyna; 2015. p. 199–208.

6. Baldes N, Schirren J. Primary and Secondary Tumors of the Diaphragm. Thorac Cardiovasc Surg 2016;64(8):641–6.

7. Akinci D, Akhan O, Mustafa O, et al. Diaphragmatic Mesothelial Cyst in Children: Radiologic Findings and Percutaneous Ethanol Sclerotherapy. Internat Rad 2004;185:873–7.

8. Karhiman G, Ozcan N, Dogan S, et al. Imaging findings and management of diaphragmatic mesothelial cysts in children. Pediatr Rad 2016;46(11):1546–51.

9. Legras A, Mordant P, Gibault, et al. Diaphragmatic bronchogenic cysts: an exceptional location. Rev Pneumonol Clinic 2014;70(6):357–61.

10. Subramanian S, Chandra T, Whitehouse J, et al. Bronchogenic cyst in the intradiaphragmatic location. Wis Med J 2013;112(6):262–4.

11. Jiang C, Wang H, Chen G, et al. Intradiaphragmatic bronchogenic cyst. Ann Thorac Surg 2013;96(2):681–3.

12. Clark FW. Subpleural lipoma of the diaphragm. Trans Path Soc Lond 1886;38:324.

13. Sampson CC, Saunders EH, Green WE, et al. Liposarcoma developing in a lipoma. Arch Pathol 1960;69:506–10.

14. Froehner M, Ockert D, Bunk A, et al. Liposarcoma of the diaphragm: CT and sonographic appearances. Abdom Imaging 2001;26(3):300–2.

15. Asahi Y, Kamiyama T, Nakanishis, et al. Chondroma of the diaphragm mimicking giant liver tumor with calcification: report of a case. Surg Today 2014;44(12):2361–5.

16. Kumbasar U, Enon S, Osman Tokat A, et al. An uncommon tumor of the diaphragm malignant schwannoma. Interact Cardiovasc Thorac Surg 2004;78(2):715–7.

17. Kumar VK, Shett S, Saxena R. Primary hydatid cyst of the diaphragm minicking diaphragmatic tumor: a case report. J Clin Diagn Res 2015;9(8):TD03–4.

18. Frederici S, Casolari E, Rossi F, et al. Rhabdomyosarcoma of the diaphragm in a 4-year old girl. Eur J Pediatr Surg 1986;41:303–5.

19. Raney RB, Anderson JR, Andrassy RJ, et al. Intergroup Rhabdomyosarcoma Study Group. Soft tissue sarcomas of the diaphragm: a report from the Intergroup Rhabdomyosarcoma Study Group from 1972 to 1992. J Pediatr Hematol Oncol 2000;22(6):510–4.

20. Strauch JT, Aleksic I, Schorn B, et al. Leiomyosarcoma of the diaphragm. Ann Thorac Surg 1999; 64(7):1154–5.

21. Blondeel PN, Christiaens mR, Thomas J, et al. Primary leiomyosarcoma of the diaphragm. Eur J Surg Oncol 1995;21. 249-231.

22. Dionne GP, Beland JE, Wang NS. Primary leiomyosarcoma of the diaphragm of an asbestos worker. Arch Pathol Lab Med 1976;100:398.

23. McCoy W. Leiomyosarcoma of the diaphragm. South Med J 1963;56:642–7.

24. Lacuna K, Bose S, Ingham M, et al. Therapeutic advances in leiomyosarcoma. Front Oncol 2023;13: 1149106.

25. Choi YS, Liu HC, Yeh TC, et al. Primary diaphragmatic yolk sac tumor and review of literature. J Pediatr Hematol Oncol 2011;33(2):e77–9.

26. Song HK, Leibold TM, Gal AA, et al. Extraskeletal osteosarcoma of the diaphragm presenting as a chest mass. Ann Thorac Surg 2002;74(2):565–7.

27. Eroglu A, Kurkcuoglu IC, Karaglanoglu N, et al. Ewing sarcoma of the diaphragm presenting with hemothorax. Ann Thorac Surg 2004;78(2):715–7.

28. Van Schil PE, Vercauteren SR, Vermeire PA, et al. Catamenial pneumothorax cause by thoracic endometriosis. Ann Thorac Surg 1996;62:585–6.

29. Marshall MB, Ahmed Z, Kucharczuk JC, et al. Catamenial pneumothorax: optimal hormonal and surgical management. Eur J Cardio Thorac Surg 2005; 27(4):662–6.

30. Augoulea A, Lambrinoudaki I, Christodoulakos G. Thoracic endometriosis syndrome. Respiration 2008;75(1):113–9.

31. Alifano M, Trisolini R, Cancellieri A, et al. Thoracic endometriosis: current knowledge. Ann Thorac Surg 2006;81(2):761–9.

32. Azizad-Pinto P, Clarke D. Thoracic endometriosis syndrome: case report and review of the literature. Perm J 2014;18(3):61–5.

33. Jubanyik KJ, Comite F. Extrapelvic endometriosis. Obstet Gynecol Clin North Am 1997;24(2):411–40.

34. Weksler B, Burt M, Bains MS, et al. Resection of lung cancer invading the diaphragm. J Thorac Cardiovasc Surg 1997;114(3):500–1.

35. Rocco G, Rendina EA, Meroni A, et al. Prognostic factors after surgical treatment of lung cancer invading the diaphragm. Ann Thorac Surg 1999; 68(6):2065–8.

36. Riquet M, Porte H, Chapelier A, et al. Resection of lung cancer invading the diaphragm. J Thorac Cardiovasc Surg 2000;120(2):417–8.

37. Yokoi K, Tsuchiya R, Mori T, et al. Results of surgical treatment of lung cancer involving the diaphragm. J Thorac Cardiovasc Surgery 2000;120(4):799–805.

38. Rusch VW. Mesothelioma and less common tumors. In: Pearson FG, Deslauriers J, et al, editors. Thoracic surgery. New York: Churchill Livingstome; 1995. p. 1083–105.

39. Fujita H, Hashimoto K, Takeda J, et al. Diaphragmatic reconstruction using a latissimus dorsi muscle flap following wide resection of the diaphragm combined with esophagogastrectomy for cardiac cancer. Jpn J Surg 1988;18:480–1.

40. Mineo TC, Biancar F. Reoperation for recurrent thymoma: experience in seven patients and review of the literature. Ann Chir Gynaecol 1996;85(4):286–91.

41. Bolukbas S, Eberlein M, Oguzhan S, et al. Extended thymectomy including lung-sparing pleurectomy for the treatment of thymic malignancies with pleural spread. Thorac Cardiovasc Surg 2009;88(3):952–7.

42. Fell SC. Surgical anatomy of the diaphragm and the phrenic nerve. In: Moores D, editor. The diaphragm. Philadelphia, PA: W.B. Saunders; 1998. p. 441–7.

43. Tanaka F, Sawada K, Ishida I, et al. Prosthetic placement of the entire left hemidiaphragm in malignant fibrous histiocytoma of the diaphragm. J Thora Cardiovasc Surg 1982;83:278–84.

44. Mishra A, Raja J, Mittal A, et al. A rare case of synovial sarcoma of diaphragm. Cancer Reports 2022; 5(9):1622.

45. Black E, Griffin S, Singh A, et al. Overview of the thorax and diaphragm and surgical anatomy of the chest wall. In: Brennan P, editor. Gray's surgical anatomy. 1st edition. Poland: Elsevier Limited; 2020. p. 294–305.

46. Rosenkratz JG, Cotton EK. Replacement of left hemidiaphragm by a pedicled muscular flap. J Thorac Cariovasc Surg 1964;48(6):912–20.

47. Furak J. Diaphragmatic reconstruction. In: Kuzdzal J, editor. ESTS Textbook of thoracic surgery. Cracow, Poland: Medycyna Praktyczna; 2015. p. 217–22.

48. McConkey MO, Temple CL, McFadden S, et al. Autologous diaphragm reconstruction with the pedicled latissimus dorsi flap. J Surg Oncol 2006;94: 248–51.

49. Finley DJ, Abu-Rustum NR, Chi DS, et al. Reconstructive techniques after diaphragm resection. Thorac Surg Clin 2009;19(4):175–80.

50. Fields BC, Ananthanaryanan V, Vigneswaran WT. A Case of Giant Primary Pleuropulmonary Synovial Sarcoma. J of Surg Onc 2020;3(4):1–4.

51. Eilber F, Dry S. Diagnosis and Management of Synovial Sarcoma. J Surg Oncol 2008;97:314–20.

52. Hitomi S, Masuda K, Kobayashi M, et al. Left Diaphragmatic Hernia After Diaphragmatic Peritonectomy for Peritoneal Cancer. J Clin Gynecol Obstet 2020;9(4):108–11.

Moving?

Make sure your subscription moves with you!

To notify us of your new address, find your **Clinics Account Number** (located on your mailing label above your name), and contact customer service at:

Email: journalscustomerservice-usa@elsevier.com

800-654-2452 (subscribers in the U.S. & Canada)
314-447-8871 (subscribers outside of the U.S. & Canada)

Fax number: 314-447-8029

Elsevier Health Sciences Division
Subscription Customer Service
3251 Riverport Lane
Maryland Heights, MO 63043

.

Printed and bound by CPI Group (UK) Ltd, Croydon, CR0 4YY

08/05/2025

01864724-0016